BACK TO
GREAT
SEX

BACK TO
GREAT
SEX

Overcome ED*
and Reclaim Lost Intimacy

═══════════

RIDWAN SHABSIGH, M.D.

Foreword by Louis Ignarro, Ph. D.

*Erectile Dysfunction

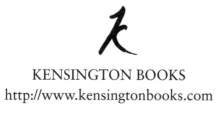

KENSINGTON BOOKS
http://www.kensingtonbooks.com

KENSINGTON BOOKS are published by

Kensington Publishing Corp.
850 Third Avenue
New York, NY 10022

All Kensington titles, imprints and distributed lines are available at special quantity discounts for bulk purchases for sales promotion, premiums, fund-raising, educational or institutional use.

Special book excerpts or customized printings can also be created to fit specific needs. For details, write or phone the office of the Kensington Special Sales Manager: Kensington Publishing Corp., 850 Third Avenue, New York, NY 10022, Attn. Special Sales Department. Phone: 1-800-221-2647.

Kensington and the K logo Reg. U.S. Pat. & TM Off.

Library of Congress Card Catalogue Number: 2001099489
ISBN 0-7582-0256-3

First Printing: August 2002
10 9 8 7 6 5 4 3 2 1

Printed in the United States of America

To my parents and family, who inspired me,
from early childhood,
to expand my knowledge and to help people in need.

To my wife and children,
who supported me throughout my professional life.

To all my patients and their partners,
whom I have had the pleasure
of helping and the privilege of interacting with.

Contents

Foreword

Erectile dysfunction (ED) is a unique health problem, because it affects millions of men; there are many misperceptions surrounding it; and men and their partners are embarrassed to talk about it. The fact that millions of men suffer from ED has motivated doctors and scientists to conduct a great amount of medical research. Scientists have always been fascinated by the fact that the penis is the only organ in the body that can generate and sustain two extremes: very high pressure during erection (almost equivalent to the top pressure in the large arteries of the rest of the body), and very low pressure during flaccidity (almost equivalent to the low pressure in the veins of the rest of the body). Everyone knew, a long time ago, that this elaborate system achieved erection and flaccidity by opening (dilation) and closing (constriction) the blood vessels and small spaces inside the erectile tissue of the penis. Furthermore, it was also clear that nerves in the penis (which are ultimately connected to the brain) controlled these blood vessels by producing small amounts of "messenger-chemicals." Scientists call these messenger-chemicals "neurotransmitters." Many years of work by our laboratory led to our discovery that nitric oxide (NO) was the principal neurotransmitter responsible for penile erection. This breakthrough in the science of medicine has opened unprecedented new avenues of research, contributing to the development of new treatments for this problem.

My journey to the 1998 Nobel Prize in Medicine started on the East Coast at the College of Pharmacy at Columbia University in New York City, and settled on the West Coast in another great institution, the University of California at Los Angeles. I am very happy to see a fellow scientist from Columbia University, Dr. Ridwan Shabsigh, make the major effort of bringing the intricate science of ED to the large number of men and their partners in clear and reader-friendly language. His book, *Back to Great Sex,* empowers men concerned with ED with the two things they urgently need: up-to-date knowledge and effective communication skills.

Louis J. Ignarro, Ph.D.
The 1998 winner of the Nobel Prize in
*   Medicine*
Professor, Nitric Oxide Research
Department of Molecular & Medical
*   Pharmacology*
University of California, Los Angeles

Preface

Sexual Health Is a Fundamental Human Right

———————•▬▬▬•———————

"There exist fundamental rights for the individual including the right to sexual health and a capacity to
enjoy and control sexual and reproductive behavior in
accordance with a social personal ethic—freedom from
fear, shame, guilt, false beliefs and other factors inhibiting sexual response and impairing sexual relationships—freedom from organic disorders, disease and
deficiencies that interfere with sexual and reproductive
function."*

In 1999, the 1st International Consultation on Erectile Dysfunction was convened in Paris to produce recommendations for
the diagnosis and treatment of erectile dysfunction (ED). This important event was sponsored by the World Health Organization
(WHO) as well as other professional organizations. More than
120 experts from all over the world thoroughly reviewed and ana-
lyzed the scientific literature and produced guidelines for the management of ED. I had the honor of participating in this conference
as a chairman of one of its committees and a member of the panel

---

*Education and treatment in human sexuality: The training of health professionals. Report of a WHO
meeting [held in Geneva from 6 to 12 February 1974] Geneva: World Health Organization, 1975. 33p.
(World Health Organization technical report series no. 572), 2.1 Definition of sexual health.

that reviewed the final recommendations. The global experts adopted and disseminated the abovementioned statement, which was based on the WHO statement from 1974 that recognizes sexual health as a fundamental human right and establishes the definition of sexual health. The following is the original source statement from 1974.

> A growing body of knowledge indicates that problems in human sexuality are more pervasive and more important to the well-being and health of individuals in many cultures than has previously been recognized, and that there are important relationships between sexual ignorance and misconceptions and diverse problems of health and the quality of life. While recognizing that it is difficult to arrive at a universally acceptable definition of the totality of human sexuality, the following definition of sexual health is represented as a step in this direction: Sexual health is the integration of the somatic, emotional, intellectual, and social aspects of sexual being, in ways that are positively enriching and that enhance personality, communication, and love. Fundamental to this concept are the right to sexual information and the right to pleasure. According to Mace, Bannerman, and Burton the concept of sexual health includes three basic elements: 1. a capacity to enjoy and control sexual and reproductive behavior in accordance with a social and personal ethic, 2. freedom from fear, shame, guilt, false beliefs, and other psychological factors inhibiting sexual response and impairing sexual relationship, 3. freedom from organic disorders, diseases, and deficiencies that interfere with sexual and reproductive functions.

Acknowledgments

Human knowledge is the fruit of collaboration and interaction. I would like to acknowledge and thank a number of persons whose input has been invaluable to this book. My brother-in-law Elbrus A. Basmouk has been a major force of support and help with the inception of this book project. Doris Rikkers provided significant help with the text, language formulation and manuscript preparation, with excellent attention to detail. Beckey Bright contributed with research, articles and summaries. Many thanks to Matt Wood for the wonderful medical art of all the figures. Thanks to Dr. Zarema Helmi for her initial medical art drafting. I would like to present my special appreciation to my literary agent Lois de la Haba, whose tireless efforts and guidance helped bring this project to a successful conclusion. Also, I would like to thank Walter Zacharius, Judy Zacharius and all the staff at Kensington Books for their excellent coordinated effort to bring this book to print. I would like to especially thank my editor Ann LaFarge for her outstanding editorial contribution. Also, many thanks to Joan Matthews for a diligent job in copyediting the manuscript.

In addition, I would like to thank all my teachers, professors, colleagues and collaborators, who shared their knowledge and experience with me and gave me intellect and inspiration. The number of persons who impressed me throughout my career could be large, but I would like to present my special appreciation to professor Peter Burchardt, the late Dr. F. Brantley Scott, Dr. Irving J. Fishman, Dr. C. Eugene Carlton Jr., Dr. Peter T. Scardino, and Dr. Carl A. Olsson.

Finally, I would like to thank all my patients and their partners and families. Their stories, experiences and outcomes have continually been enriching my knowledge and enhancing my research and education.

Introduction

As a young boy I dreamed of becoming a pilot. Everything about airplanes—their shape, design specifications, and even the noise—was fascinating to me. What attracted me most to flying was the continuous innovation and discovery that pervaded that field.

But then everything changed—my brother gave me a biology kit that contained a microscope. Overnight I turned from an aviation enthusiast to a biology fanatic. With biology and medicine I combined my love for innovation and discovery with my desire to help people in need, which ultimately led me to pursue medical school and a career as a doctor. My career in a top academic institution (Columbia University) and its teaching hospital (the New York Presbyterian Hospital), in the specialty of urology and sexual dysfunction, combines my love for continuous innovation and discovery with the ability to help a large number of people. These two great things have become part of my daily life.

Scientists involved in sexual dysfunction research are continuously making new discoveries regarding how organs and tissues function during sexual activity. Such discoveries have involved the vascular system (blood vessels), the central and peripheral nervous systems, hormones and ultimately the genes. New diagnostic methods and innovative treatments have been the hallmark of this field of medicine. For example, after years of successful treatment with penile self-injections, medical therapy for erectile dysfunction has seen the introduction of an effective and safe oral pill, Viagra®. Extensive research continues to investigate other oral medications, some of which are in the later stages of clinical trials and may be on the market very soon. Discovery and innovation are an intimate part of my professional life, and have permeated my personal goals from the beginning.

The pleasure I get from helping people is a large part of what drives me in my work. Many men and women suffer from a variety of sexual dysfunctions that can lead to a reduction of quality of life, depression, stress, and relational conflicts. The majority of them suffer in silence because of embarrassment, ignorance, or lack of access to medical professionals who can help them. Helping those men and women to get back to great sex is one of my most professionally gratifying experiences.

Educating the patient and frequently the patient's partner about the nature of sexual dysfunction, its causes and risk factors, goes a long way in helping a couple. I spend a lot of time explaining and educating my patients and other physicians about sexual dysfunction, its causes and treatments. Through this book I hope to reach millions more people who are in desperate need of information to calm their anxiety and to encourage them to seek professional help. I receive great joy and fulfillment when I realize that a treatment for a patient's dysfunction has been effective and continues to provide him with successful and satisfying sex.

Another highly successful and gratifying aspect of my approach to this field of medicine is my comprehensive diagnostic and treatment approach, including all physical and psychological factors. Traditionally, some treatments have emphasized the physical nature of the disorder, while others have addressed only the psychological issues. I believe that man is a seamless, nonseparable combination of the physical and the psychological, or body and soul. Conducting my practice with this comprehensive approach not only helps more patients and their partners, but also increases the quality of care. Sexual dysfunctions are not like other medical conditions. They often involve issues of identity and self-worth, and frequently impact not only the patient, but also his relationships with others.

Recognizing how many men are affected by erectile troubles, however, is only the beginning of the battle. Besides being much more prevalent than scientists first believed, erectile dysfunction is also widely undertreated. Many men and their partners falter at the thought of seeking help: they are embarrassed and humiliated. Compared with other societies, America is still relatively bashful about sex. Most people do not want to share their sexual problems with strangers, and thus an overwhelming majority of men refuse to seek a medical professional. Because so few men actually come forward with their problem, it is difficult to put an exact figure on the extent of erectile dysfunction, but it is estimated that less than 25 percent of men with erectile disorders seek medical help. And while the introduction of Viagra® has increased the percentage of men seeking treatment from about 5 percent to around 25 percent, this still leaves 75 percent of men untreated!

Privacy is very important to people who are faced with any medical issue, and even more so when the condition is a sexual and a highly personal one. My patients come to me with all sorts of excuses for delaying or avoiding treatment. Many are embarrassed; others are frightened. These feelings and situations are often painful and destructive, for many men and their partners, but they are not necessary. Years of hearing stories from patients who, in seeking help, have felt violated, ostracized, or targeted have convinced me that information and knowledge about the subject of healthy sexual performance and where to seek help when their sexuality is hindered will prevent more patients from feeling this way. The best patients work with their doctors in finding the best remedy for restoring their sex life. This book is based on the valuable concept of educating you and assisting you in finding a reputable doctor who will explain treatment options and help plan a course of action. My foremost mission, which I hold dearest, is to give you as much up-to-date information as possible in a simple and easily comprehensible way. Education and understanding, combined with the correct facility, can work wonders for bringing the goal of getting back to great sex within anyone's grasp.

QUESTIONS MY PATIENTS ASK

Q: My husband and I know we haven't had great sex (any sex, really) for a long time, but we don't really know what our problem is. Is it me? Him? Both of us? How do we begin restoring our sex life?

A: The first step is to open the line of honest and clear communication between you and your husband about this problem. Continuing to build on the open communication leads to clear understanding of ED and collaboration between you and your husband on solving this problem. The next step is to seek the professional advice of a doctor. Restoring great sex to your life or your lives is a process and not a onetime deal. It is important to follow through after the initial visit to the doctor.

Q: Sexual dysfunction seems to be a very complicated medical subject. Where should I start looking for information?

A: There are a number of sources for information. The library certainly has numerous health books. Although there might not be many books such as this one, dedicated to the subject of erectile dysfunction (ED), most health books have sections on sexual health and sexual dysfunctions including ED. The Internet also is a good source of information. [See a list of informational websites at the end of this book.] Keep in mind that your doctor is an excellent source of information and education. He or she can give you information and also help you sort out the overwhelming and sometimes confusing data on the various topics related to ED.

Q: My doctor does not seem to have enough time to answer my questions about ED. What can I do?

A: Doctors nowadays function under tremendous pressure by managed care to see as many patients as possible and spend as little time as possible with each individual patient. Although most doctors would love to spend time educating their patients and answering their questions, the reality of managed care and HMOs makes this very difficult. However, there are a few things that you can do. First, if you are seeing a primary care physician, try to schedule an appointment dedicated to discussing ED. Trying to seek help for ED in the course of a doctor's visit for other reasons, e.g., annual checkup, high blood pressure care, diabetes follow-up, might overcrowd the visit with too many medical issues, thus preventing you from getting the information you need about ED. If your primary care physician is not available to spend time with you on your ED, request a referral to a specialist—a urologist or, preferably, a urologist known to take care of ED as a subspecialty. Try to educate yourself about ED as much as you can prior to your doctor's visit: read about ED, write down your questions, and be prepared with personal information. When you're with your doctor, be sure to take notes of the conversation and any recommendations.

I

Stop Making Excuses

The first step in getting back to great sex is simple—stop making excuses. Problems in the bedroom, whether physical or psychological, whether male or female, thrive on silence. Stop the excuses and rationalization. Start communicating—with your partner and your doctor—to get on your way back to great sex.

But let's face facts: Good sex requires a penis that functions correctly, that can achieve and maintain a firm erection. Sexual encounters require an erect penis. Without this, sex is definitely dysfunctional, and that's why it is important for us to focus on erectile dysfunction first.

Erectile dysfunction (ED) is like an unwanted guest in any household. It can show up unexpectedly or gradually make its presence known. Most middle-aged men know it's around, as if it were a bogey man lurking in the closet or under the bed—ready to strike. They live in dread of it and come up with a myriad of excuses for its existence. But excuses are as bad as silence. ED thrives on silence. The problem only exacerbates itself when it is ignored. And making excuses to yourself or to others (if you do dare to mention ED) only makes things worse.

Every time I interview a new patient, I ask a standard question: "How long have you had this problem?" And almost without fail, I am astonished to hear that my patient has put up with ED for months, years, even decades. He's come up with all types of excuses for not discussing his most intimate problem with his doctor.

I've heard every possible excuse and reason you can imagine. And you know what? There really is *no excuse*. There are many ways to regain sexual function. Few patients leave my office feeling that there's nothing that can be done for them. There is hope, no matter what the cause.

Let me share with you some of the excuses I've heard over the years. Perhaps one of them is yours.

It doesn't really matter.

Let me first say, it *does* matter. Your sexual dysfunction can diminish and complicate your life. It can lead to a reduction in the quality of life, depression, frustration, and stress and cause conflicts in your relationships and in your job. If you were in constant pain from a knee injury to the point that you had difficulty walking, wouldn't you seek help? You would know almost immediately that your dysfunction would limit your life: you couldn't walk around Disney World, you couldn't go dancing on Saturday nights with your wife, you couldn't walk the golf course as you used to, and your tennis days would be over. Your quality of life would be lowered and you would go and get help. Just because your knee is not as personal as your penis doesn't excuse you from talking to your doctor.

I'm too old.

Just because you're getting older does not mean you have stopped desiring or enjoying sex. Sex is generally desirable, enjoyable, and quite common even among those of advanced age. Although age is the most proven risk factor for ED, it is not inevitable that you have to stop having sex just because you've turned 50 or 60 or even 80. Sometimes ED moves in on the coattails of other unwanted guests of the aging body: diabetes, high blood pressure, stress, depression, and heart disease. It can also result from long-standing bad habits: smoking, alcoholism, or use of illegal drugs. But none of those factors, or your age, should stop you from seeking help to restore great sex.

Maybe it will go away.

No, ED won't go away on its own. As I told you, it thrives on silence. It may show up silently for good cause, but if you ignore it, it won't just vanish overnight. It'll creep deeper into your mind, spoil your relationships, and steal your contentment. Ignoring it won't make it go away—it will only complicate the matter.

It will be better when I'm not so stressed about work.

Stress has a way of affecting many aspects of your life, and ED can show up arm-in-arm with stress. But if your stress eases and ED is still around, you'd better make a call to your doctor.

It must be my high blood pressure medication.

It is true that many medications can affect your sexual function, and your high blood pressure may also be at fault. But either way, you don't have to live with the ED. Call your doctor, and explain the problem. He might be able to adjust the dosage of your medication or change your prescription. Either remedy can alleviate your ED. Whatever you do, don't stop taking your high blood pressure medication. Work with your doctor.

It's my partner's fault.

Ah, now here's a complicated problem. Although your partner may not enjoy sex as much as before, owing to her age and changes in her body, she is not the cause of your ED. If your relationship is strained in some way, your partner is not the cause of your problem. You need to seek professional help to find out the underlying reason for your sexual problem, whether it be from a medical doctor, a marriage counselor, or both. You can work this out with open and honest communication. In most cases the cause of ED is complicated with several contributing factors.

I just need to relax.

Stress, anxiety and depression can affect your performance, but if the problem continues, even after a long relaxing weekend, or the stressful event is long past, you need to call your doctor.

I need a vacation.

Sorry, but ED will come along with you on a vacation. Just like a persistent untreated cough or indigestion doesn't stay behind when you leave for Hawaii, neither does ED.

I'm probably just drinking too much.

Although alcohol has some effect on sexual function, it usually takes prolonged and excessive drinking to damage the nervous system to the extent that ED results. An occasional glass of wine with dinner will not necessarily adversely affect your sexual function.

It's all in my head.

Chances are it's not. Very few cases of ED are solely psychologically based. But check it out. What might really be a physical problem can soon also become a psychological one.

All I need is Viagra®.

Maybe, maybe not. No doubt Viagra® seems like the answer for every problem in the bedroom, but sorry, it's sometimes not as simple as popping the little blue pill. Call your doctor; he or she is the one best qualified to diagnose your problem. Viagra® will be at the top of the list if your doctor knows it will help you. But there are some very good reasons for not prescribing Viagra®, so follow your doctor's advice.

It's too embarrassing to talk about.

Most people find very personal things embarrassing to talk about. Most people don't want to discuss money matters honestly unless they are talking to their financial adviser or their broker—

they are usually embarrassed to admit how much (or little) they are worth. The same is true with our sex lives. But you should be comfortable talking about this private part of your life with a professional—your doctor.

I don't know whom to ask.

Start first with your primary care physician. He or she will be able to help you or direct you to a specialist. Otherwise, check the listings at the end of this book to get you started in finding the help you need and deserve.

So, which excuse do you like to use? By now you realize that there are no excuses and no simple answers. Your sexuality is complex. And when you have a problem, there's usually not just a simple solution like rest or a vacation or a prescription for Viagra®. Your body doesn't work independently from your brain, and in turn, both of them don't work apart from your interactions with other people.

"Sex is not only an erection, and relationship and love are not only sex" is a wise statement. Sexual dysfunction affects you as a whole person: your mind, your body, your self-esteem, and your partner. Your best treatment will come when you realize you need to treat the whole self, not just one part.

Drop the excuses. Stop procrastinating. It's time to educate yourself so you are ready to ask intelligent questions of your doctor, discuss your feelings with your partner, and get back to great sex.

II

Getting to Know ED

If you're like most healthy, normal males, you've become pretty used to your penis and its reliable performance by the time you're middle-aged. So when you occasionally encounter ED face-to-face through nonperformance or a less than rigid erection, you may panic. Don't. It's very normal that occasionally the stress of life, overwork, a case of the blahs, or a bout with the flu may hinder a stellar performance in bed. So before you run off to your doctor for the latest wonder drug, review these definitions of ED and get to know a little more about it.

DEFINITIONS OF ED

"Erectile Dysfunction is the consistent or recurrent inability of a man to attain and/or maintain a penile erection sufficient for sexual performance" (1st International Consultation on ED, sponsored by the World Health Organization, July 1999).

"Erectile Dysfunction is the persistent or repeated inability, for at least 3 months duration, to attain and/or maintain an erection sufficient for satisfactory sexual performance" (Process of Care Consensus Guidelines Panel, December 1997).

"Erectile Dysfunction is the inability of the male to attain and maintain erection of the penis sufficient to permit satisfactory sexual intercourse" (National Institutes of Health Consensus Development Conference on Impotence, December 1992).

It's okay and perfectly normal if you occasionally experience erectile dysfunction, but if the experience becomes a regular occurrence for more than 3 months, you probably should check in with your doctor. And don't feel bad, or ashamed or embarrassed. *You are not alone.* Scientists have discovered that ED is much more common than they ever expected, and because risk increases with age, they expect its prevalence to escalate as the male population continues to grow older. They estimate that about 10 to 20 million men suffer from ED and that up to 30 million men in the U.S. alone experience at least partial loss of function. Statistics for the world are even more staggering. Estimates of men experiencing ED run as high as 152 million worldwide. With the growth and aging of the world population, it is expected that the number of men with ED will even rise to 322 million in the year 2025.

> *ED is different from other sexual disorders such as premature ejaculation, anorgasmia (lack of orgasm), or lack of sexual desire. However, ED may occur at the same time as these other problems.*

Erectile dysfunction has been around for a long time, but it was the ailment that no one wanted to admit to or talk about. Everyone assumed it happened only to "old" men. At the turn of the last century, life expectancy was much shorter for the average male than it is right now, so few men even faced the problem, or they felt they could live without this sexual aspect of their lives. However, at the beginning of the twentieth century there was a tremendous interest in the hormonal aspects of sexuality. Hormonal treatments with testicular extracts or later with testosterone remained prevalent among practitioners for almost a hundred years. We now know that pure hormonal causes of ED are uncommon and that testosterone treatment is required only for men whose lab reports prove they have low testosterone.

In the late 1960s, the majority of medical textbooks stated that the most common causes of ED were psychological. Sometimes, unspecified psychological causes were credited for ED, other times a variety of psychological factors such as performance anxiety, stress, sexual identity problems, and relationship conflicts were named. In the 1970s researchers were able to verify and measure naturally occurring nocturnal erections. Once the measurement system was in place, they were able to confirm that these spontaneous nighttime erections were *not* present in men who suffered from ED as a result of physical causes.

Then in the 1980s, with the discovery of the anatomy and physiology of the vascular system of the penis, doctors shifted their attention to the organic (physical) causes of ED. At that time doctors believed that the majority of patients with ED had organic causes such as diabetes, vascular disease, high blood pressure, high cholesterol, and hardening of the arteries (arteriosclerosis). Psychological factors suddenly became less significant.

Research in the 1990s based on the U.S. male population confirmed organic causes or risk factors in relationship to ED. The 1990s, however, also introduced serious research in the field of psychology and the relationship of depression to ED as well as the importance of a couple's relationship: romance, intimacy, communication, and love and how that interacts with ED. The phrase "erectile dysfunction" was first used and recommended in 1992 by a committee of the National Institutes of Health as a preferred term rather than the word "impotence." Impotence is a pejorative term that may include a variety of sexual dysfunctions (loss of libido, orgasmic or ejaculatory dysfunction) whereas "erectile dysfunction" specifically refers to erectile disability and implies a medical condition.

TIME LINE

Ancient times	ED considered a myth.
1694	J. van Musschenbrack in Leiden, Netherlands, describes experiments with vacuum air pumps to treat ED.
1874	John King (American) uses vacuum device in a clinic setting.
1889	Brown-Sequard (French) injects himself with testicular extract.
1900	Cause of ED thought to be hormonal.
1934	Bogoras (German) implants rib cartilage into the penis as a "natural implant."
1946	After World War II, beginning of the Baby Boom.
1948	Alfred Kinsey reports on ED based on a survey of volunteers.
1950s–1960s	Cause of ED thought to be psychological.
1952	First penile implants described, using acrylic prosthesis.
1965	Last year of the Baby Boom.
1970s	Penile implants become a popular treatment for ED.
1970s	Doctors turn their attention to organic (physical) causes of ED owing to the study of nocturnal erections.
1973	First inflatable penile prosthesis implanted.
1980s–2000	Remarkable amounts of information, knowledge, and advances in the field of ED.
1980s	Causes of ED thought to be organic (physical) because of interest in vascular causes and better understanding of penile anatomy and physiology.
1982	First report that an erection can be achieved by injecting papaverine into the penis.
1987–1989	First Massachusetts Male Aging Study conducted.
1990s	Causes of ED classified as organic, psychological, or mixed.
1992	National Health and Social Life Survey (NHSLS) performed to inquire into U.S. sexual practices and beliefs in young adults.

1992	National Institutes of Health define erectile dysfunction during its first consensus development conference on impotence.
1992	Pfizer researchers stumble on a medication (later known as Viagra®) that causes erections as a side effect.
1994	MMAS estimates the number of men with ED in the United States at 30 million.
1995	FDA approves the use of prostaglandin E_1 alprostadil sterile powder (Caverject® manufactured by Upjohn, now Pharmacia) penile self-injections for treatment of ED.
1995	Number of men with ED worldwide is estimated at 152 million.
1995–1997	Follow-up survey conducted on Massachusetts Male Aging Study (MMAs).
1996	First of the Baby Boomers turn 50.
1996	FDA approves the use of prostaglandin E_1 alprostadil intraurethral suppository (MUSE® manufactured by Vivus) for treatment of ED.
1997	FDA approves the use of prostaglandin E_1 alprostadil alfadex (Edex or Viridal manufactured by Schwarz Pharma) penile injections for treatment of ED.
1998	FDA approves the first effective and safe oral medication: sildenafil (Viagra®) for treating ED.
1998–2000	The percentage of patients with ED seeking treatment expands, as compared to pre-1998, but the majority of men remain untreated.
1999	1st International Consultation on Erectile Dysfunction held in Paris. Sponsored by the WHO.
1999	Research to develop new treatments of ED expands to develop new oral medications, topical gels, and even gene therapy.
2000	Twenty-first century focuses on the importance of relationships, emphasizing issues of romance, intimacy, communication, and love.
2000	Rising interest in male aging, including male andropause.

April 2000	FDA approves Androgel as a treatment for male hypogonadism or testosterone deficiency.
January 2001	The European Drug Review Agency (the equivalent to the FDA) recommends the approval of Uprima® (sublingual apomorphine) for the treatment of ED.
June 2001	Following positive results on its new oral drug Cialis™, Lilly-ICOS submits the New Drug Application to the FDA.
September 2001	Following positive results on its new oral drug Vardenafil, Bayer submits the New Drug Application to the FDA.
2010	Male population of the world over age 50 will exceed 670 million.
2015	Last of the Baby Boomers turn 50.
2025	Number of men with ED worldwide is projected to be 322 million.

Now, at the beginning of a new century, we are far ahead of where we were a hundred years ago, and yet we are also back where we started in the last century—talking about and investigating the role hormones play in sexuality. Talk of "male menopause" or "andropause" is becoming more popular as the population ages. Each of these approaches to ED over the last century has been correct, but only partially. Now it's evident that all of these various approaches must be considered in order to create a total and comprehensive method of treatment.

ED is a common and significant medical problem. Doctors now agree that about 80 percent of all erectile dysfunction has primarily a physical rather than a psychological cause. So if you were worried that it was all in your head, think again.

The medical profession classifies ED as:

• Organic (physical): due to vascular (blood vessels), neurological (nerves), hormonal, or cavernosal (chambers inside the penis) abnormalities.
• Psychogenic: due to mental, behavioral, or emotional problems when no organic cause is found.
• Mixed: a combination of organic and psychogenic causes.

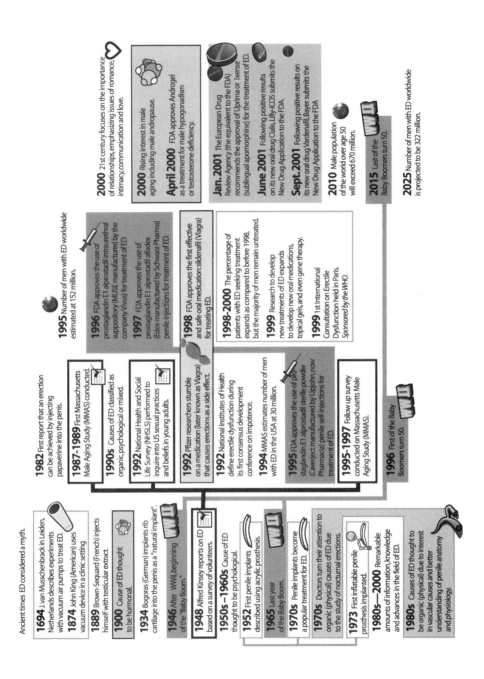

Figure 1. Time line of the development of the sciences of erectile dysfunction and related issues.

CAUSES OF ED*

1. Certain treated diseases: diabetes, high blood pressure, heart disease, high cholesterol, kidney disease.
2. Certain medications.
3. Cigarette smoking.
4. Excessive alcohol consumption.
5. Suppression/expression of anger.
6. Depression.

*According to the Massachusetts Male Aging Study.
(See Chapter III for more information.)

ED also has various levels of severity depending on the ability to achieve and maintain an erection:

- Minimal: usually achieve and maintain an erection but rigidity varies.
- Moderate: sometimes achieve and maintain an erection.
- Complete: never achieve or maintain an erection.

SELF-RATING QUESTIONNAIRE*

How would you describe your ability to get and keep an erection that is rigid enough for satisfactory sexual activity?

A. *No ED*
   Always able to get and keep an erection good enough for sexual intercourse.
B. *Minimal ED*
   Usually able to get and keep an erection good enough for sexual intercourse.
C. *Moderate ED*
   Sometimes able to get and keep an erection good enough for sexual intercourse.
D. *Complete ED*
   Never able to get and keep an erection good enough for sexual intercourse.

*With permission: Massachusetts Male Aging Study, New England Research Institute.

STUDIES ON ED

Only three population-based studies about erectile dysfunction have been published. Alfred Kinsey (the Kinsey report) polled volunteers from northern Indiana and the Chicago area regarding their sexuality in 1948. Since most volunteer studies are biased (those most interested in a subject being surveyed volunteer) the Kinsey report findings can only be taken as suggestive and are not reliable enough to use in long-term comparison studies.

The Massachusetts Male Aging Study (MMAS) was a survey conducted to study the prevalence of ED with increased aging. This study was a random-sample observational survey of 1,709 noninstitutionalized men, ages 40 to 70, conducted from 1987 to 1989 in communities in and near Boston. Trained interviewers collected data by interviewing men in their homes. The data included a self-administered sexual activity questionnaire, physiological information, demographics, socioeconomics, psychological indices, health status, medications, lifestyle, smoking habits, alcohol consumption, and blood samples. ED was classified as minimal, moderate, and complete. Response rate to the survey was excellent at 75 percent. This survey used modern probability sampling techniques. It is especially valuable because of the follow-up survey done some eight years later on 1,156 participants of the first survey.

The third significant study on sexuality was the National Health and Social Life Survey (NHSLS) conducted in 1992. It was a national probability survey of 1,410 men and 1,749 women between the ages of 18 and 59 years of age, living in households (not colleges, jails, or other institutions) throughout the United States. The sample completion rate was greater than 79 percent. This survey accounts for about 97 percent of the population in this age range—roughly 150 million Americans. The NHSLS obtained information about the sexual practices and beliefs among younger adults in the United States, whereas the MMAS focused on erectile dysfunction in aging males. The surveys nicely complement one

another, and where their findings overlap, the information is re-
markably consistent.

It is from these three significant studies of sexuality that all
statistics and information about ED is extracted. Data from these
three studies show that the risk of developing erectile problems is
strongly associated with aging. The Massachusetts Male Aging
Study showed very clearly that ED was highly prevalent with 52%
of the sample of men 40–70 years old reporting ED (see Figure 2).
Age was the strongest correlate of both the total prevalence of ED
and the prevalence of complete ED. At age 40, the total prevalence

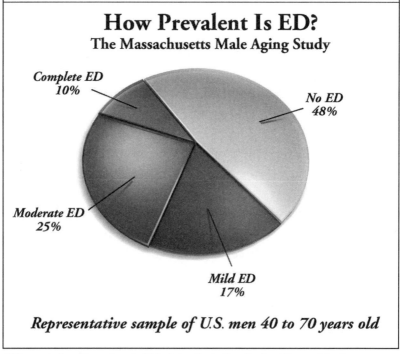

With permission: Massachusetts Male Aging Study, New England Research Institute.

Figure 2. This pie graph from the Massachusetts Male Aging Study shows how common ED
is. Approximately half of all men aged 40 to 70 years have some degree of ED, and 10 percent
have complete ED.

of ED was 39% and the prevalence of complete ED was 5%. At age 70, the total prevalence of ED was 67% and the prevalence of complete ED was 15%. In all age groups, minimal ED remained the same, but the moderate and complete categories increased with age. This suggests that ED is a progressive condition. As men grow older, their organs age as well, and they become more susceptible to illnesses that can lead to ED. Even the medications needed to treat those illnesses can limit sexual function (see Figures 3 and 4).

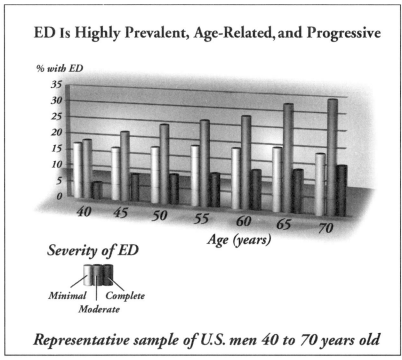

With permission: Massachusetts Male Aging Study, New England Research Institute.

Figure 3. This column graph from the Massachusetts Male Aging Study shows that the occurrence and severity of ED increase with age.

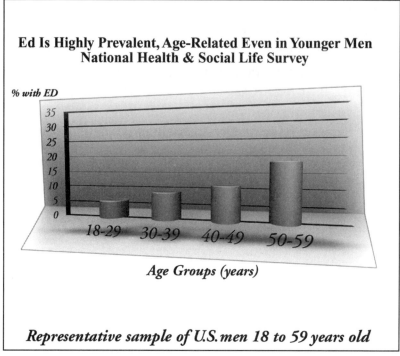

**Ed Is Highly Prevalent, Age-Related Even in Younger Men
National Health & Social Life Survey**

Representative sample of U.S. men 18 to 59 years old

With permission Lauman et al. JAMA 281:537–544.
Copyrighted 1999 by The American Medical Association.

Figure 4. This column graph from the National Health & Social Life Survey shows that even in a young age range of 18 to 59 years, the occurrence of ED increases with age, with a sharp increase after age 50.

SUCCESSFUL AGING

Since the Baby Boomers are growing older and becoming a significant part of the world's population, doctors are more determined than ever to ensure this age group not only an extended lifetime, but also a high quality of life, including the continuation of great sex. This view of aging has been called "successful aging." Those over 50 are seeking their doctors' advice and treatment for the major health conditions that accompany aging: erectile dysfunction, benign prostatic hyperplasia, cardiovascular disease, and depression. As a result, researchers are trying to learn more about these health problems and how to prevent and treat them in order to maintain the highest possible quality of life for the patient.

Successful aging has three aspects:

1. Decreasing the likelihood of disease and disease-related disabilities.
2. Maintaining high mental and physical capacity.
3. Continuing to participate in life activities.

Successful aging involves combining all three elements; although each, taken separately, is important, it is their combination that completely conveys the concept of successful aging. In finding a treatment or therapy for any health problem, you and your doctor should consider not only whether or not it will cure you, but also if it will make you happy and increase the quality of your life. Treatment for treatment's sake is no longer good enough; treatment needs to ensure physical health as well as overall well-being.

Growing older brings with it a gradual physical decline. Although you can try to slow down the process by eating right and staying physically fit, your body parts will start to slow down—and that includes the sex organs as well. You should not, however, be alarmed at these gradual changes—they are perfectly normal.

Normal aging signs related to sexual function are:

1. It takes longer to achieve an erection.
2. Stronger stimulation is needed to achieve an erection.
3. Erection is weaker and of shorter duration.
4. It takes longer to achieve a second erection.
5. Spontaneous erections occur less frequently.

Since ED is age related, doctors are beginning to believe that it might be wise to screen all men over age 50 for erectile dysfunction. Some statistics say that by age 50, approximately half of all men experience some degree of ED, and in the year 2000, every 15 seconds another man turned 50! Now for the good news—there is still the other 50 percent of men over 50 who do *not* have erectile dysfunction. Some men remain sexually active, with no problems, even into their eighties or nineties.

BUT DO I REALLY HAVE ED?

Since many men are concerned about their sexual function and want a quick-and-easy way to find out if there is a problem, the 1st International Consultation on ED sponsored by the World Health Organization at the conference in July 1999 came up with the questionnaire given below. This questionnaire is called the ED Intensity and Impact Scale. (You may see it again in your doctor's office.) The quiz consists of six questions: five are to detect ED and to determine its intensity, and one is to discover how ED has affected you. The five-item intensity scale was based on extensive research and clinical experience. It is highly reliable and valid and has been translated into more than thirty languages. Your total score will be useful in diagnosing and establishing the severity of your erectile dysfunction.

You can take this test at home in complete privacy, but be sure to share your findings with your doctor if and when you need the help of a professional.

ED INTENSITY SCALE*

Each question has several responses. Circle the number of the response that best describes your own situation. Please be sure that you select one and only one response for each question.

Note: *The following questions should be completed only by men who have been sexually active and have attempted sexual intercourse in the past 3 months. For sexually inactive men, the questionnaire may be answered for the last period of time (3 months or longer) during which the individual was sexually active.*

1. How often were you able to get an erection during sexual activity?

Almost never or never	1
A few times (much less than half the time)	2
Sometimes (about half the time)	3
Most times (much more than half the time)	4
Almost always or always	5

2. When you had erections with sexual stimulation, how often were your erections hard enough for penetration (entering your partner)?

Almost never or never	1
A few times (much less than half the time)	2
Sometimes (about half the time)	3
Most times (much more than half the time)	4
Almost always or always	5

*With permission: *Erectile Dysfunction,* 1st International Consultation on ED cosponsored by the World Health Organization (WHO), International Society of Impotence Research (ISIR), and Societe Internationale d'Urologie (SIU). Edited by A. Jardin, G. Wagner, S. Khouri, F. Giuliano, H. Padma-Nathan, and R. Rosen. Health Publications Ltd., 2000.

3. When you attempted intercourse, how often were you able to penetrate (enter) your partner?

Almost never or never	1
A few times (much less than half the time)	2
Sometimes (about half the time)	3
Most times (much more than half the time)	4
Almost always or always	5

4. During sexual intercourse, how often were you able to maintain your erection after you had penetrated (entered) your partner?

Almost never or never	1
A few times (much less than half the time)	2
Sometimes (about half the time)	3
Most times (much more than half the time)	4
Almost always or always	5

5. During sexual intercourse, how difficult was it to maintain your erection to completion of intercourse?

Extremely difficult	1
Very difficult	2
Difficult	3
Slightly difficult	4
Not difficult	5

Instructions for scoring: Add the scores for each item 1 through 5 (total possible score = 25). ED severity classification: total score 5–10 (severe ED); 11–15 (moderate ED); 16–20 (mild ED); and 21–25 (no ED or normal).

ED IMPACT (DISTRESS OR BOTHER) SCALE*

If you were to spend the rest of your life with your erectile condition the way it is now, how would you feel about that?

Very dissatisfied	1
Rather dissatisfied	2
Mixed, about equally satisfied and dissatisfied	3
Rather satisfied	4
Very satisfied	5

Your internist or primary care physician will *not* be shocked if you mention you are having sexual problems. But then again perhaps he or she will be surprised since the medical community estimates that more than 75 percent of men with erectile dysfunction do not seek medical help! Don't be one of them.

> *Of the estimated 30 million men in the United States with ED, only 7 million were treated in the 3 years following the introduction of Viagra®. Of the 152 million men worldwide with ED, only 14 million were treated: ED remains undertreated.*

You don't have to accept erectile dysfunction and less than great sex as your lot in life, no matter what your age. Your doctor can help you determine what options are available and which treatments are right for you and your partner. (More about that later.) Treatments continue to improve as scientists investigate the human body and better understand the physiology and anatomy of an erection. There's lots of hope.

---

*With permission: *Erectile Dysfunction,* 1st International Consultation on ED cosponsored by the World Health Organization (WHO), International Society of Impotence Research (ISIR), and Societe Internationale d'Urologie (SIU). Edited by A. Jardin, G. Wagner, S. Khouri, F. Giuliano, H. Padma-Nathan, and R. Rosen. Health Publications Ltd., 2000.

QUESTIONS MY PATIENTS ASK

Q: Is erectile dysfunction the same as impotence?

A: Yes. Impotence was the common term used until the National Institutes of Health (NIH) consensus development conference in 1992. That conference recommended replacing the term "impotence" with erectile dysfunction (ED). The World Health Organization's (WHO) first international consultation on ED in 1999 repeated the same recommendation. ED is a more accurate medical term with less negativity than "impotence." My patients use a variety of terms to communicate their ED: "I can't get a hard-on." "My erections aren't firm enough." "I lose it too quickly." "I can't perform." "My nature is shot." "My penis is weak." "I can't make love." "I can't penetrate." "It doesn't last."

Q: I'm 30 years old. I've never had a "miss." I've always had a "hit." Last weekend, to my great shock, it took a lot of effort to get an erection; and when I got one, I lost it very quickly! Do I have ED? Or am I developing ED?

A: Don't panic! Having one miss or a few times of having difficulty getting and maintaining an erection does not mean you have ED or that you are developing ED. Many men experience short periods of sexual difficulty. This might be caused by physical or psychological factors such as illness, fatigue, stress, or too much alcohol. The WHO guidelines recommend at least a period of 3 months of erectile difficulties to qualify for a diagnosis of ED. If you experience erection difficulties for 3 months or longer, seek help from your doctor.

Q: Does ED go away?

A: In most patients, ED is irreversible, especially those who have diabetes, vascular disease, multiple sclerosis, injuries, and pelvic surgery. However, in patients whose ED is caused by psychological or hormonal factors or is a side effect of medication,

ED may be reversible. A full evaluation by your doctor, or a referral to a specialist, will help you determine the prognosis of your ED. (For more on this subject, see the Afterword, "Preventing ED.")

Q: *Is it appropriate to get treatment for ED at any age, regardless of how old I am?*

A: Yes. As long as you have adequate sexual desire, you are physically and mentally reasonably healthy, and you would like to enjoy sex, it's appropriate to get a medical evaluation and treatment for ED, even at an advanced age.

Q: *My interest in sex is moderate and I would enjoy it, but I'm not sure about the sexual interest of my wife/partner. Should I still seek help?*

A: It's surprising how many couples don't communicate openly about sex and their sexual desires and concerns. Remember, not communicating doesn't necessarily mean not caring. Open up the lines of communication with your partner. You might be pleasantly surprised by how much your partner cares about sex and about having a satisfactory sexual relationship with you.

Q: *My partner and I don't talk about sexual issues and definitely not about my ED. What should I do?*

A: When it comes to ED, there are numerous reasons for a lack of communication: embarrassment, shyness, ignorance, fear of hurting the other's feelings, and misperceptions. Simply take the first step and begin a warm, caring, and honest conversation. If the start proves to be difficult, a psychologist or a sex therapist might help facilitate communication and interaction.

Q: *I do not need a doctor! All I need is Viagra®! Should I order it over the Internet?*

A: No! ED might be associated with risk factors that relate

to other important health conditions such as diabetes, high blood pressure, or hormonal deficiency. A full evaluation by a doctor is very beneficial. Buying Viagra® over the Internet will deprive you of the benefit of a detailed interview by a doctor, a physical examination, and lab tests. The Internet does not replace the direct and personalized interaction between the doctor and the patient.

III

The Physical and Psychological Causes of ED

The word "dysfunction" means that something doesn't work right. Something has gone wrong. But in order to understand what's going wrong, let's first review what happens when everything is going right and an erection comes on naturally.

With rare exception, all males are born with a penis that knows exactly what to do naturally. Even as an infant you occasionally (much to the surprise of your mother) had an erection. As a toddler and preschooler you discovered that it was comforting and exciting to "make that little fellow stand up." As you reached puberty, erections occurred spontaneously at night or during masturbation. And as a young adult you took your sexual ability for granted, since, without fail, an erection occurred at the appropriate (or even inappropriate) times.

Erections in a male are natural and normal. Erections are actually vital for maintaining a healthy penis. Researchers have observed that penile muscle cells deprived of oxygen start to accumulate collagens that eventually cause scar tissue. Providing the penis with a regular supply of fresh, oxygen-rich blood, such as that which flows to the penis during an erection, prevents the accumulation of these harmful collagens. In this way, nocturnal erections may be nature's way of counteracting this process.

What causes an erection is basically very simple: An erection is the result of an increased flow of blood into the penis and a decreased outflow. An erection is a reflex reaction caused by mental or physical stimulation or both. When the male is sexually aroused, nerve messages from the brain begin to release chemicals that increase blood flow into the penis. Blood enters the penis faster then it exits, thus causing an erection to take place. The erectile tissues of the penis, or the twin chambers, are called the corpora cavenosa (see Figure 5). The corpora cavernosa are smooth muscles made up of lacunar spaces (tiny vascular spaces that contain in their walls smooth muscle cells). These two chambers act like one because the wall or partition that separates them is incomplete. The corpora cavernosa or erectile tissues accept blood as quickly as a sponge might soak up water, giving them the unique ability to trap the blood and allow the penis to swell and become rigid. When the corpora cavernosa begin to dilate, they exert pressure on the outgoing veins that would normally expel the blood. Due to the pressure, the veins are closed off, the corpora cavernosa remain filled with blood, and the erection is maintained. After a man climaxes, the blood leaves the penis and the erection quickly subsides (see Figure 6).

That sounds simple enough. So what can go wrong?

In the heat of a passionate moment, I'm sure you're not thinking of how all these body parts, from your brain on down, are working. But each function must work just right in order for an erection to occur and to be maintained.

Let's start with an early step—the one about the brain sending nerve messages to release chemicals. The chemicals that convey messages from the nerves are called neurotransmitters, which make the blood vessels in the penis relax or open up. Some of the chemicals that cause relaxation of the smooth muscle tissues in the penis, and consequently allow an erection to occur, are nitric oxide, prostaglandin E_1, and vasointestinal polypeptide.

Along with these chemicals, there is an opposing group that

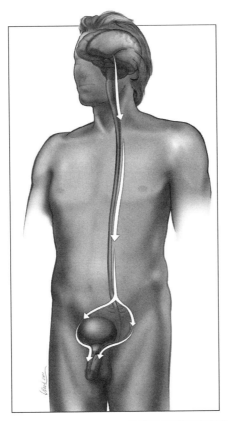

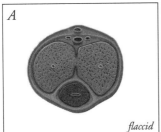

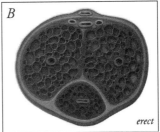

Figure 5. How erection and flaccidity occur. Sexually stimulating incoming signals from fantasy, touching, seeing, and smelling are processed in various parts of the brain ending in processing centers in the midbrain and the hypothalamus. In addition, signals from direct stimulation of the genital area are processed in the spinal cord in the lower back. The brain and spinal cord send nerve signals to the vascular structures of the penis to create an erection. The insets [A and B] show cross-sections of the structures of the penis, including the two erection chambers or the corpora cavernosa. A: In the flaccid state, the arteries are constricted and the lacunar spaces are collapsed and empty. B: In the erect state, the arteries and the lacunar spaces are dilated and filled with blood.

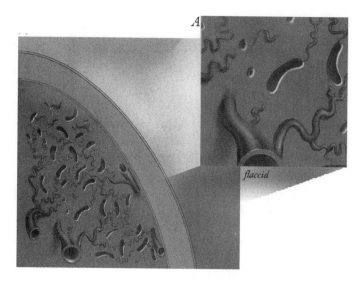

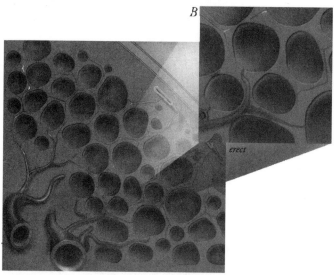

Figure 6. This illustration shows, in higher magnification, what happens in the erectile tissue of the penis. The corpora cavernosa are made up of lacunar spaces, which are tiny vascular spaces. A: In the flaccid state, the lacunar spaces are collapsed and empty; the arteries are constricted and the veins are open. B: During erection, the corpora cavernosa, or erectile tissues, accept blood like a sponge, giving them the unique ability to trap the blood, and allow the penis to swell and become rigid. When the corpora cavernosa begin to dilate, they exert pressure on the outgoing veins that would normally expel the blood. Due to the pressure, the veins are closed off, the corpora cavernosa remain filled with blood, and the erection is maintained. After a man climaxes, the blood leaves the penis and the erection quickly subsides.

causes the smooth muscle to constrict, thus narrowing the blood vessels in the penis. When the blood vessels are contracted, the penis becomes flaccid. This group of chemicals, or neurotransmitters, include adrenaline and noradrenaline.

The balance between how open or closed the blood vessels are in the penis determines how rigid or flaccid the penis becomes.

> *Smooth muscle relaxation = vasodilation = erection*
>
> *Smooth muscle contraction = vasoconstriction = flaccidity*

Now let's talk a little more about the nerves. When a man is sexually stimulated, either physically or mentally, two nerve pathways are activated. The first pathway causes a reflex erection through the sacral spinal cord (the lower end of the spinal cord). No connection to the brain needs to occur, which explains why a man with a spinal cord injury is often still capable of producing some degree of an erection. The second nerve pathway occurs between the brain and the multitude of nerves within the penis. This center sends messages down the spinal cord to the erection center in the lower spinal cord. From the spinal cord, the signal travels through the peripheral nerves to the corpora cavernosa of the penis. These nerve cells create nitric oxide, which causes the penis to form a chemical called cyclic guanosine monophosphate, commonly referred to as cyclic GMP or simply cGMP (see Figure 7).

> *The discovery of nitric oxide as the chemical that dilates blood vessels throughout the body (not just in the penis) was the reason that three American scientists—Dr. Louis Ignarro, Dr. Robert Furchgott, and Dr. Feride Murade—won the Nobel Prize for Medicine in 1998.*

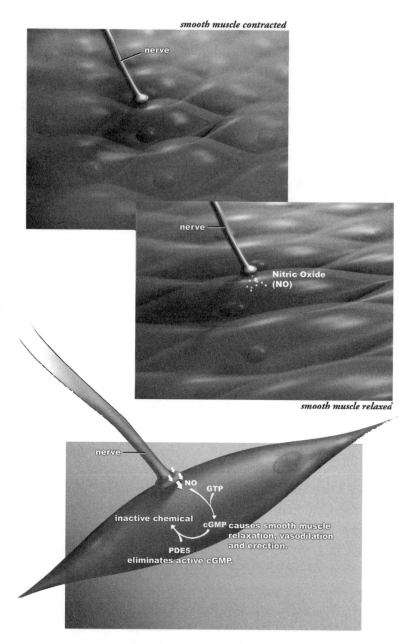

Figure 7. This illustration shows the junction of a nerve and a smooth muscle cell inside the walls of the lacunar spaces of the corpora cavernosa. Upon sexual stimulation, the nerve end produces the signaling chemical or neurotransmitter nitric oxide (NO). This produces cGMP, which causes smooth muscle relaxation, vasodilation, and erection. cGMP is continually converted by PDE-5 to an inactive chemical.

Cyclic GMP dilates (opens and broadens) the blood vessels within the penis, allowing it to engorge with blood. The result is a rigid and erect penis. In normal circumstances, a man continues to produce abundant amounts of cGMP for the duration of the sexual act. Simultaneously, another chemical known as phosphodiesterase 5, or PDE-5, diminishes the effects of cGMP and creates an equilibrium in the erectile tissue. Ultimately, this balancing act allows the erection to continue.

Once a man's sexual arousal dies down, or stimulation stops, cGMP production comes to a halt. With PDE-5 as the predominant chemical, the penis returns to its flaccid state.

Okay, so maybe it's all more complicated than that opening definition. But now you realize that many systems of the body are involved in an erection: the brain, chemicals, spinal cord, blood vessels, and the nervous system. Everything needs to be in working order and performing together to make a successful and sustaining erection.

When one system is not in perfect working order owing to disease, medication, or injury, an erection may not occur as expected.

There are three basic physical mechanisms that can cause erectile dysfunction:

1. Failure to Initiate
   With this neurological problem, the nerve messages from the brain or the spinal cord do not reach the penis to get the process of an erection started. Diabetes, multiple sclerosis and spinal cord injury may cause this problem. Injuries or surgery to the pelvic area such as radical prostatectomy for treatment of prostate cancer can damage the penile nerves.

2. Failure to Fill
   In this vascular problem, not enough blood flows into the penis through the blood vessels to make it rigid. There are many conditions that can reduce the blood

flow into the penis, causing erectile dysfunction. The most common problem is hardening of the arteries (arteriosclerosis). Diabetes, high blood pressure, high blood cholesterol, and cigarette smoking can also cause hardening of the arteries and thus erectile dysfunction. Traumatic injuries such as a fall onto the crossbar of a bike or a pelvic fracture from a car accident might also cause reduced blood flow.

3. Failure to Store

   In this situation a man is unable to attain or maintain an erection because the penis is unable to store the blood. Instead the blood leaks out, thus the problem is called "venous leak." This "end organ disease" is frequently caused by advanced atherosclerosis, diabetes, or fibrosis (scar tissue formation) of the corpora cavernosa.

PHYSICAL CAUSES OF ED

ED that is caused by a physical problem will come on slowly. You may gradually realize that your ability to attain or maintain an erection is poor or that your penis is not as rigid as it used to be. In contrast, a problem that is psychological in nature may suddenly show up during intercourse and yet you will have normal erections in the morning or during masturbation.

DISEASES THAT ARE ASSOCIATED WITH ED

1. Diabetes

   This disease can cause nerve damage (neuropathy) and damage to the circulatory system, specifically to the blood vessels that supply the penis. Healthy nerves and blood vessels are critical for producing an erection. More than 50 percent of diabetic males have erectile dysfunction.

2. Vascular disease
   Arteriosclerosis (hardening of the arteries)
   Hypertension (high blood pressure) and high cholesterol both affect blood flowing in and out of the penis. This is usually the most common physical cause of ED.
3. Heart disease: coronary artery disease or heart attack.
4. Nerve diseases: including spinal cord injury, multiple sclerosis, or nerve degeneration due to diabetes or alcoholism; or complications resulting from prostate, bladder, rectal, or colon surgery.
5. Kidney disease.
6. Stroke, particularly if the left side of the brain is involved.

SURGERY AND TRAUMA

Any major injury or surgery to the pelvic area can cause damage to the nerves and/or blood vessels leading to the penis. Spinal cord injuries; injuries resulting from a fall, car accident, or biking accident; surgery for colon, rectal, or prostate cancer; and even radiation therapy in the pelvic area can cause damage to nerves and blood vessels that may result in ED.

DRUGS THAT CAUSE ED

Common medications can also be a cause for erectile dysfunction. There is a long list of prescription drugs and over-the-counter medications that have the side effect of causing ED. Allergy (hay fever) medicines, high blood pressure medicine, and illicit drugs such as marijuana, cocaine, and heroin are all well-known causes of ED. If you notice a change in your sexual function shortly after starting a new medication, you should visit your doctor and ask about a possible connection between the two.

Let me make one thing clear, however: Many of the diseases you take medication for are in themselves causes for ED (see the list above). Never stop taking any medication without first consulting your doctor. Your life is at risk if you stop taking the medication that controls your high blood pressure, your heart disease, or your arteriosclerosis.

Drugs frequently associated with ED. (This is a partial list. Check with your doctor about these and other medications in your individual case.)

1. Antihypertensives (used to treat high blood pressure)
   Thiazide diuretics, beta-blockers
   Common drug names: Hydrochlorothiazide, Aldactone®, Inderal®
2. Antidepressants (used to treat depression and anxiety)
   Tricyclic antidepressants, selective serotonin reuptake inhibitors (SSRIs)
   Common drug names: Anafranil®, Prozac®, Zoloft®, Paxil®
3. Antiarrythmics (used to treat irregular heartbeat)
   Digoxin
   Common drug name: Digoxin, Lanoxin®
4. Antiandrogens (used to treat prostate cancer)
   Common drug names: Lupron®, Zoladex®
5. H2 Blockers (used to treat ulcers)
   Cimetidine
   Common drug name: Tagamet®
6. Over-the-counter medications
   Antihistamines (used to treat hay fever): Sudafed®
7. Other drugs
   Propecia® (for hair loss prevention)
   Proscar® (for reducing the size of an enlarged, noncancerous prostate gland)

8. Recreational drugs
   Marijuana, cocaine, heroin, methadone, ecstasy
   Chronic and prolonged use of these drugs causes nerve damage and affects the ability to attain and maintain an erection.

Your doctor will do all he or she can to treat your cardiovascular disease or depression with medications that do not interfere with your sexual function. However, caring for these primary diseases must take priority over your ED. Thus, if the most effective drug for your heart disease or depression interferes with your erection ability, you might choose the effective therapy for your heart disease or depression and pursue an additional therapy for your ED. (Don't worry; there are many options. See Chapter V.)

LIFESTYLE OPTIONS THAT CAUSE ED

Alcohol has both an immediate and long-term effect on sexual function. Heavy drinking immediately reduces your ability to have a strong erection. Long-term, excessive drinking can cause neuropathy (nerve damage). It might also affect the liver and the hormonal system.

Men who *smoke* are twice as likely to suffer from ED.

**SEXUAL MEDICINE SOCIETY
OF NORTH AMERICA, INC.**

Position Statement:
Smoking and Erectile Dysfunction

Cigarette smoking is a risk factor for erectile dysfunction. Men who smoke have a greater chance of developing erectile dysfunction compared to men who do not smoke.

A sedentary lifestyle can affect your love life. Men who sit around, watch TV and don't exercise also have a tendency to overeat and overdrink—all of which are bad for your general and sexual health.

RISK FACTORS

The following conditions or habits are major risk factors for ED. Which ones are present in your life?

Diabetes

High blood pressure

High blood cholesterol levels

Heart disease: heart attack, bypass surgery

Blood vessel disease (hardening of the arteries)

Stress

Depression

Anxiety

Accidents causing injury to the pelvic area or penis

Surgery to the genitals or groin area

Heavy alcohol consumption

Cigarette smoking

Drug abuse (cocaine, marijuana, or heroin)

Sedentary lifestyle

Even if you do not have any of these risk factors, there is one thing that you can't stop with medication, exercise, or lifestyle change: that's aging. If you are over 50, chances are you may encounter ED just because you are getting older. Men of 50-plus years may often lose reliable erectile function owing to a subtle decline of their sex drive. They are entering a time of less efficient sexual functioning. Simply getting older may be the cause of your ED, not heart disease or hypertension or any special medication. Patience, understanding, and open communication with your partner and your doctor are the first steps in the treatment of ED at any age.

PSYCHOLOGICAL CAUSES OF ED

Although physical and medicinal problems can often be the culprit for the first occurrence of nonperformance, your psyche kicks in almost immediately and complicates things. That first time that you can't initiate or maintain an erection may start you on a negative thinking, downward spiral leading to a more complex situation. That's why I encourage you to check with your doctor as soon as you suspect something. Your initial problem may just be the new high blood pressure medicine or even the dosage—both of which are easy for your doctor to adjust. Or maybe it's hay fever season and your prescription medicine has made your waking hours more comfortable, but your time in bed very uncomfortable. Try to approach the situation rationally and immediately. There may be a very simple solution to your ED, but if you don't talk about it to your partner and your doctor and just keep thinking it will go away, the problem will fester and grow in your mind, creating an even bigger problem to contend with later.

For years during the 1950s and 1960s most doctors thought the primary cause for ED was psychological. Facts now prove that that is not true. In older men (40 years or older) more than 80 percent of cases are physical (diabetes or hardening of the arteries) or medication-related. But in most cases, there are multiple factors contributing to ED. Sometimes the physical, psychological, and chemical are all mixed together. If the problem were simple, the solution would be simple. But humans aren't simple and neither are most of their problems, so most solutions for ED are usually quite complex.

Sexual activity requires the mind and the body working together. Emotional or relational problems can cause ED or worsen it. Depression; stress at home or work; marital conflicts; relational problems with family, friends, or co-workers; and anxiety about your sexual performance can all contribute to ED and its severity.

As I have said before, the body and the mind work together to generate sexual activity. Consequently, emotional and relational problems can cause or worsen ED. Almost everyone has a psychological reaction to ED even if the primary cause is a physical one. Men with ED or low sexual desire experience a general decrease in their quality of life, including a perception of low physical satisfaction, low emotional satisfaction, and low general happiness.

Purely psychological reasons for the occurrence of ED are uncommon. Of the 30 million men estimated to have ED, less than 10 percent had solely a psychological cause of this problem. Occasionally psychological problems are deep seated in an individual, having accumulated since early childhood. It is best to seek the help of a mental health professional in dealing with any significant psychological problems causing ED.

With most cases of ED, however, there is some psychological aspect to the onset or continuation of this dysfunction. Rarely is ED caused purely by a physical (organic) or purely psychological (functional) reason. There is usually a combination of the two. If at some time in your adult life you have had adequate erectile function, and now are unable to perform, this is called Acquired Psychogenic Erectile Dysfunction. Erectile dysfunction can affect your self-esteem, coping ability, and social and occupational performance; therefore this problem cannot be ignored. Depression, stress at home or work, marital conflicts, job loss, sexual orientation maladjustment, relational problems with your sex partner, anxiety about sexual performance, anxiety in general, suppressed anger, and past or present abuse whether physical, emotional, or sexual can all affect your sexual performance.

Depression and ED are a bit like the riddle, "Which came first, the chicken or the egg?" Most men are well aware that erectile dysfunction may cause depression, but it has also been scientifically proven that depression can cause ED. The psychological effects of ED—depression and anxiety—are well known. Just like most failures in life (job loss, divorce, unrealized aspirations), sexual failure can result in depression. Men with ED are more likely to be depressed and have a decreased sex drive. Depression due to occurrences of erectile dysfunction may hinder sexual performance, create further depression, and eventually lead to avoiding all sexual contact. Men who are depressed usually have a lower sex drive, no longer find pleasure in things they once enjoyed, such as sex, and also have ED. Men who suffer from depression and ED are also more likely to discontinue treatment for their ED than those with ED alone.

Some doctors believe that both depression and ED are the result of ADAM: Androgen (hormones) Decline in the Aging Male. Symptoms include:

1. Decreased sex drive and sexual function
2. Changes in mood: an increase in depression or anger
3. Decline in lean body mass; and increase in body fat
4. Decreased body hair
5. Decreased bone density

These changes are due to a decline in the production of testosterone that occurs as you get older. The decrease in the testosterone levels leads to a decreased sex drive as well as ED and depression. But it really doesn't matter whether ED leads to depression or depression results from ED: these two conditions usually show up hand in hand in most aging men and require attention and treatment.

Recent research suggests that two questions are sufficient for knowing if you have depression.*

1. *During the past month, have you often been bothered by feeling down, depressed, or hopeless?*
2. *During the past month, have you often been bothered by little interest or pleasure doing things?*

If you answer yes to these questions, be sure to bring it up with your doctor. You do not need to feel this way; it is not natural and it might not "just go away." Talking to your doctor about how you feel will help him help you.

*Wooley, M.A. et al. Journal of General Internal Medicine, 1977, 12:439-49.

Extreme levels of anger, either suppressed (you keep it all inside) or expressed (you rant, rave, and throw things) are associated with the occurrence of ED. In fact 75 percent of men with extreme anger also have ED: twice that of those with average anger levels. To the best of my knowledge, no studies have yet been conducted on the relationship between anger and ED; however, anger has a way of "eating away" at the mind and body, causing ulcers, high blood pressure, and mental instability.

Your relationships with others, both negative and positive, can affect your emotional well-being. There is also a wide range of topics that can contribute to a psychological aspect of your ED. Review this list. Use it as a tool to help you express to your doctor what factors in your emotional life may be contributing to your problem.

Preexisting factors
   Restrictive upbringing
   Disturbed family relationships
   Inadequate sexual information
   Traumatic early sexual experiences
   Past sexual abuse
   Early insecurity in psychosexual role
Contributing Factors
   Depression
   Caring for a newborn
   Unreasonable expectations
   Dysfunction in your partner
   Failure in other areas of life
   Discord in the general relationship
   Reaction to organic factors
   General anxiety
   Traumatic sexual experience
   Guilt feeling
Maintaining Factors
   Performance anxiety
   Depression

Guilt

Inadequate sexual information

Psychiatric disorder

Unhappiness in the general relationship

Loss of attraction between partners

Fear of intimacy

Low self-esteem, poor self-image

Restricted foreplay

Sexual myths

Poor communication

Just remember that the more information you can give your doctor—which, by the way, will be held in strict confidence—the better he or she can analyze your situation, alleviate your dysfunction, and restore your sexual well-being.

QUESTIONS MY PATIENTS ASK

Q: Is the penis a muscle?

A: The penis is not a muscle in the sense of other muscles that move parts of the body, such as muscle in your arms and legs. But, scientists report, there are "smooth muscle cells" in the erectile tissue of the penis. These are the cells that actively open up the blood vessels (dilate) to fill the penis with blood and create an erection, or close the blood vessels (constrict) to empty the penis and create flaccidity. (See Figures 6 and 7, pages 36 and 38.)

Q: How does an erection happen?

A: Erection is a neurovascular event. Stimulation, by touching, seeing, smelling, and fantasizing, will be transmitted to the central nervous system via the sensory nerves. The brain and the spinal cord will process this stimulation input and generate orders via the motor nerves to the blood vessels to open up (dilate) and fill the penis under high pressure. (See Figure 5, page 35.)

Q: I cannot have a second or a third erection, like I used to. Do I have ED?

A: Young men are frequently capable of having two or more erections and orgasms in one sexual encounter. With age, this capability is normally expected to decrease. If you are capable of having one satisfactory erection and orgasm without difficulty, most probably you do not have ED.

Q: Why does diabetes cause ED?

A: Diabetes causes malfunction of the nerves and blood vessels in the body. The body depends on the nerves and the blood vessels to generate an erection. Therefore, a disease like diabetes, which damages the nerves and the blood vessels, is logically expected to cause ED.

Q: My ED started when my internist prescribed a pill for my high blood pressure. Should I stop taking it?

A: No. Leaving high blood pressure untreated could be dangerous and might cause complications such as stroke, heart failure, or kidney failure. Check with your doctor and ask about your alternatives. Your doctor might change your blood pressure medication. If changing medication does not help your ED, continue the medication to control your blood pressure and ask your doctor for a way to treat the ED.

Q: I feel that the cause of my depression is my environment. I need to solve my family problems and reduce my work stress. Why should I discuss depression with my doctor?

A: Although your problems with your family or work will contribute to depression, depression is also partially caused by internal factors in the central nervous system. Regardless of the cause, depression is frequently associated with ED and might complicate treatment. In addition, depression is associated with increased risk for cardiovascular disease. It also might cause difficulty in handling the demands of everyday life. You should openly discuss all issues related to depression with your doctor.

Q: What caused my ED? Is it important to know the cause?

A: The cause of your ED might be one or more of the risk factors/causes listed and discussed in this chapter. In certain cases, the cause of ED is very clear, such as pelvic surgery (radical prostatectomy, radical cystectomy, removal of the rectum) or trauma, such as spinal cord injury or pelvic fracture. In other cases, it might be unclear, occurring in a 48-year-old, otherwise healthy man. Knowing the cause might not change the treatment of ED in many patients, because many treatments (such as oral pills, injections, and implants) are not cause-specific. However, detecting the cause of ED in an individual patient frequently has the advantage of realizing the risk factors and addressing important lifestyle issues such as exercise, weight, and smoking, as well as partner relationship and communication.

Q: I read somewhere (or my doctor told me) that the cause of ED in the majority of patients is related to hardening of the arteries (arteriosclerosis). Since I have ED, am I at risk for diseases of the heart and blood vessels, such as coronary artery disease, heart attack, and stroke? Should I get a cardiology checkup?

A: The most common cause of ED is vascular disease. ED patients frequently have other cardiovascular conditions, such as a history of heart attack, hypertension, and diabetes. But there is no need for panic. Look at the onset of ED as an opportunity to take a break from your busy life, think about your lifestyle, and ask yourself some questions. Do I exercise enough? Do I smoke? Am I overweight? Do I drink too much alcohol? Do I use illegal drugs? If I'm a diabetic, do I keep my blood sugar under control? If I have high blood pressure, do I keep my blood pressure under good control? How do I handle stress? Do I overwork? Do I think I might be depressed? How is my relationship and communication with my partner? Do I have a family history of heart disease? Or more ominously, do I have chest pain or shortness of breath? Consult with your doctor. Your doctor will advise you, based upon the answers to some of the above questions, whether you need to see a heart specialist.

IV

What Happens in the Doctor's Office

If you're getting ready to visit your doctor, you need to know what to expect when you get there. But let me first congratulate you on taking this step. Many men never make this move—in fact, 75 percent of men who suffer from ED never seek treatment! It's unfortunate that they don't, for no one needs to live with ED. Besides that, it's of the utmost importance for you to see your doctor, not only to find a way to restore your sexual performance, but also to review your general health.

One of the critical things you should look for, expect, and require of your doctor is that he address the multifaceted aspects of ED. I strongly believe in, and use, a comprehensive approach to patient care. It would be inappropriate for your doctor to just give you a prescription for Viagra® over the phone without first gathering information. Let's go through the steps of what would happen in my office, as if you were my patient. First I would request that you complete a form giving me your name, address, phone number, age, education, etc. I would also ask you to fill out a form with your complete medical history.

Not until you're in the privacy of my office will I ask you anything personal about your sexual medical history. Many of my

---

DO'S AND DON'TS FOR SEEING YOUR DOCTOR

Do's:	Don'ts:
Be open.	Don't be embarrassed.
Be honest.	Don't fear judgmentalism.
Be prepared with information.	Don't hold back anything.
Offer specifics.	Don't stifle your feelings.

---

patients are embarrassed, avoid eye contact, and are very vague about their sexual problem, finding it hard to hear themselves speak words relating to their sexual anatomy or function. Please be reassured that your doctor is working for you. Perhaps if you are more aware of the type of information he or she is looking for, you will be more confident and comfortable about expressing yourself. Most doctors have seen it all and heard it all. They have studied extensively and are very familiar with the human body as well as human emotions.

Your sexual history will include the details of your sexual problem or problems, explaining the nature, onset, duration, severity, and surrounding circumstances of your condition. It is necessary for you to express exactly what your problem is. Some men have difficulty describing the exact nature of their problem. In addition to ED, there are various problems within the category of sexual dysfunction:

- *Problems with libido:* low sexual desire
- *Problems with ejaculation:*

  Rapid/premature ejaculation is the occurrence of ejaculation before or very soon after the beginning of intercourse (before or within 30 seconds of the beginning of intercourse).

  Delayed ejaculation: undue delay in reaching a climax during sexual activity.

  Absence of ejaculation during orgasm: anejaculation.

  Retrograde ejaculation: backward passage of semen into

the bladder after emission, usually due to the bladder neck mechanism failing to close. Sperm will appear in the urine after orgasm.

• *Problems with reaching orgasm:* inability to achieve an orgasm during conscious sexual activity (anorgasmia).

• *Problems with erection:* the consistent or recurrent inability of a man to attain and/or maintain a penile erection sufficient for sexual performance. (This is what we've been focusing on.)

These problems may be present with or without ED. It is very helpful for your doctor to know exactly what the nature of your problem is since there are different treatments for each one. Familiarize yourself with these terms so you can clearly communicate with your doctor.

If you have had any previous diagnostic tests or treatments, I record those too. Then I will discuss with you your goals and expectations. Next I will complete, with your help, a review of your past medical, surgical, psychological, and social history, as well as listing your medications, habits (smoking, drinking, recreational drugs), relationships, partner history, physical activity level and tolerance. Finally I'll give you a physical exam. Although you may feel that this gathering of information is an invasion of your privacy, I need to know all the details regarding your life in order to successfully treat you with a methodology that will personally appeal to you and work with your lifestyle.

Once I have all this information, I can give you a diagnosis. I may ask you to undergo some additional tests, including lab tests; if not, I'll discuss treatments with you and may recommend counseling for you and your partner while you start on medication. We'll discuss your options for treatment. If you have any questions or concerns, I'll give you plenty of time to discuss them.

Let me give you an example of how this complete awareness of a patient works.

Larry, age 55, came to me complaining that he had been having problems attaining and maintaining erections for about a year.

His medical history revealed that his diabetes of the last seven years had been under control until about two years ago, when he had accepted early retirement from his employer. Following his early retirement, Larry gradually became depressed. This led him back to his habit of smoking, which he hadn't done for several years. He stopped exercising and started eating junk food, thus causing him to gain weight. The increase in weight, in turn, raised his blood sugar and lipids and he developed high blood pressure.

Larry's relationship with his wife declined as his depression grew. They argued constantly. The beginning of erectile dysfunction became the last major blow to Larry's already shaken self-confidence and self-esteem. He felt inferior to his wife because he was retired and she was still working as a teacher. His feelings of inferiority were magnified with the ED.

As Larry shared all that information with me, I realized that there were a number of intertwined organic, psychological, and interpersonal factors involved in his problem. Larry's body and mind were involved in his ED. Diabetes, high blood pressure, high blood lipids, smoking, and his sedentary lifestyle all were risk factors for ED from the organic side. Depression and marital conflict were risk factors from the psychological side. I knew I couldn't fix just one aspect of this problem: Larry and I needed to address all these issues in a systematic, comprehensive approach to give him not only a satisfactory sex life, but also physical and psychological well-being, and general happiness as well.

My first step was to explain to Larry this combination of risk factors. I told him I wanted to treat him with what I call a parallel approach—treating several aspects of his problem at the same time. I gave him a prescription for Viagra® to address his ED, and encouraged him to make some lifestyle changes: stop smoking, lose weight, and exercise. Simultaneously I referred him to an internist to get his blood sugar and blood pressure under control. I also referred him to a psychiatrist, who started Larry on a low dose of an antidepressant.

Larry's wife was willing to help in any way she could to support her husband, so she became involved in the process right away. I adjusted Larry's office appointments to fit his wife's schedule and invited her to come to all of his visits, which she did. This was a great opportunity for her to learn the medical information firsthand and for them as a couple to have a forum in which to communicate about their sex life and any other relationship issues.

Although Viagra® was the medication of choice for Larry, its effectiveness was not consistent for him. After discussing it at one of our appointments, Larry, his wife, and I decided on self-injection therapy with Caverject® (see page 99). This treatment was very effective, successful, and satisfying for Larry and his wife. Ultimately, he used Viagra® and Caverject® alternately. Through the course of treatment addressing the various aspects of ED, Larry and his wife regained their self-confidence, developed better communication skills, achieved happiness, and returned to great sex. They even started exercising together. Larry lost some weight, gained control of his blood sugar and blood pressure, and successfully quit smoking. This case really had an impressive outcome!

INITIAL EVALUATION INFORMATION

1. *Sexual history*
2. *Medical history*
3. *Psychosocial history*
4. *Physical examination*
5. *Lab tests*
6. *Diagnosis*
7. *Patient questions/education*
8. *Treatment or referrals to a specialist*

Let's now review each part of the evaluation information in more detail, so you are prepared to answer questions and provide information for your doctor. (See "Fill This Out and Take It to Your Doctor" at the back of this book. This form can save you and your doctor time and help you organize your thoughts prior to visiting your doctor.)

SEXUAL HISTORY

If you're like most people, discussing your sex life may be difficult and embarrassing. I just want to reassure you that your doctor is only seeking this information to help you. He or she will protect your privacy and keep everything strictly confidential. Remember that the goal is to reestablish your sexual well-being, and your doctor is the key to helping you get there.

You'll also be asked questions about the nature and chronology of your problem, the psychosocial context, the severity, and what your needs and expectations are. Here are some questions you may be asked to establish that information.

Nature/Chronology
1. Can you describe your sexual problem?
2. When was the last time you had a satisfactory erection?
3. How was your sexual function prior to this time?
4. Was the onset of your dysfunction gradual or sudden?
5. When was the last time you had satisfactory penetration?
6. What portion of sexual attempts is satisfactory to you?
7. Is your partner satisfied with your sexual function?
8. If we can restore your erections, what would be your average frequency of sex each month?

Severity/Quantity
1. Do you have morning or nighttime erections?
2. How strong are the erections you get with masturbation?
3. On a scale of 1 to 10, with ten being normal, how would you rate the stiffness of those erections?
4. With sexual stimulation can you initiate an erection?

5. With sexual stimulation can you maintain an erection?

6. Do you lose erection before penetration, or before climax?

7. Do you have to concentrate to maintain an erection?

8. Do you lose the erection if you don't have continuous direct stimulation to the penis?

9. Is there a significant bend in your penis? Or any other change in shape?

10. Do you have pain with erection?

11. Do you have difficulty reaching orgasm?

12. Do you have problems with ejaculating too soon or not at all?

Desire/Partner Issues

1. How strong is your desire for sex, now and in the past?

2. Is your erectile problem related to your partner or a certain situation?

3. Is your partner able to become aroused when you have sex together?

4. What has been your partner's reaction to your sexual difficulties?

Another questionnaire that would help you explain your sexual difficulty to your doctor is the "ED Intensity and Impact Scales" on pages 27–29. Let your doctor know if you have filled it out and what the results are.

WHAT TO BRING TO THE DOCTOR'S OFFICE

1. A list of all the medications and the dosages you are currently taking.

2. Copies of the completed forms from the back of this book, or the information that is contained on those forms.

MEDICAL HISTORY

This will include a checklist of diseases such as diabetes, high blood pressure, heart disease, etc. You'll be asked to list any surgery you have had and the dates. Be sure you're aware of your childhood diseases, injuries, and surgeries as well as recent ones. You may also be asked to supply information about the health of your parents and siblings. You'll be asked if you smoke, drink, or take recreational drugs and to list any prescriptions you are currently taking. For this last one, you should make a list before you leave home so you know the exact name and dosage of each medication you take. Be sure to also include any vitamins and herbs you consume regularly.

PSYCHOSOCIAL HISTORY

Different doctors will handle this information in different ways, but what they are seeking is information about your general well-being and lifestyle. You may be asked to answer questions such as the following:

How old are you? How many years of education do you have? How are you feeling about your life in general? Are you depressed, feeling overly anxious, or under extreme stress? Have you recently experienced any major changes or losses in your life? How do you view yourself and your self-worth? What is your relationship with your partner(s)? Are you happy with your current employment? Have you ever been sexually abused?

PHYSICAL EXAMINATION

This exam is not substantially different from your yearly physical; however, it does focus more on the genital-urinary system, as well as the vascular (blood vessels) and neurological (nerves) systems. Feel free to ask your doctor what he is looking for as he checks your blood pressure (vascular system) and your penis and testicles (genital-urinary system). He will also perform a rectal exam to check the prostate gland. Any pain in the prostate may make sexual activity uncomfortable.

To evaluate the nerves in the penis, your doctor may check to see if there is enough feeling in the area around your penis. He may also check your bulbocaverosus (BC) reflex by squeezing the glans of your penis. These exams are all very routine and are not painful. They are, however, critical for an accurate diagnosis of your ED.

LAB TESTS

Basic blood and urine tests will be required to measure your testosterone and other hormone levels as well as lipid levels. A low testosterone level may cause ED and other sexual dysfunctions. Blood lipid levels reveal if there is a risk of hardening of the arteries. A fasting blood sugar test checks for diabetes. These basic routine tests are valuable for understanding your overall general health.

DIAGNOSIS

In some cases the diagnosis is very clear and your doctor will communicate it to you in the first visit. In other cases there is not just a quick fix for the problem of ED, so your doctor may not have a full diagnosis available for you on your first visit. He or she will probably ask you to stop by again after the results of any lab tests have come in. In the diagnosis, your doctor will review all the information you have provided, present you with the facts, and explain your options for treatment.

PATIENT QUESTIONS/EDUCATION

On your first visit, be sure your doctor takes the time to answer your questions and give you information.

Some of my patients want as much knowledge and information about ED as possible. Others just want me to take care of it so they can get back to "normal." I usually go over several items with my patients to make sure that they completely understand:

1. The anatomy and physiology of male sexuality
2. The causes, common risk factors, and lifestyle contributors of ED
3. The results of the physical exam and any basic lab tests
4. The need, in some cases, for additional specialized tests
5. What they expect from the treatment
6. All options of treatment
7. The multistepped nature of treatment
8. The importance of ongoing communication to successfully restoring their sexual health

All this information may not come in the first visit. It may be communicated throughout two or more visits, depending on the nature of the situation. I prefer to give my patients as much information as they can handle on the first visit and then encourage them to read up on the topic, review what we've talked about, and come back to go over any additional questions they may have or clarify something that was not completely understood in our first discussion. Communication between doctor and patient is critical throughout the entire treatment process.

TREATMENT OR REFERRAL TO A SPECIALIST

At this step your doctor may be ready to recommend a treatment or to refer you to a specialist in the field of urology, endocrinology, psychiatry, sex therapy, or counseling. But only the minority of cases need referral to a specialist. Most primary care physicians are now capable of handling ED effectively especially since the introduction of oral medications. If, however, you feel uncomfortable with your physician, be sure to request a referral to a specialist, who may make you feel more comfortable in talking about and treating your sexual dysfunction.

SPECIALIZED TESTS

When your doctor needs to know the specific reason for your ED, or needs more information in order to know how best to treat your ED, he or she will probably suggest that you undergo some additional tests. Some cases of ED require these extensive tests. Keep in mind that there is no perfect test. Each diagnostic test has limitations. Your doctor will be most qualified to help you understand the detailed features of each test. Here are a few of the tests that your doctor might request.

Nocturnal Penile Tumescence and Rigidity Test (NPTR). This test takes place in the comfort of your home over two to three consecutive nights and measures the number of erections, or lack thereof, you have during deep sleep. Erections during sleep are a natural process that occurs two to five times at night, if there is no physical reason to prevent them. If the test shows normal erections occurring while you sleep, your doctor may explore the possibility of a psychological reason for your ED. If normal erections do not occur, your doctor will consider the possibilities of a vascular, hormonal, or neurological problem.

The common technique for testing NPTR is the RigiScan® method. The RigiScan® is a mechanical device capable of constantly measuring the circumference and rigidity of the penis throughout the night. The device consists of a recording piece of equipment that is secured to your thigh. It's connected to two sensor rings that are placed around the base and near the tip of the penis (see Figure 8). The RigiScan® can collect data for up to 10 hours at a time and records the circumference and rigidity of the penis and the duration of each erection. After two or three consecutive nights of gathering data, you bring the device back to the office. The data is then downloaded into a computer and printed out on a graph, which your doctor will be able to interpret for you (see Figure 9).

Vascular Testing

Intracavernosal Injection Test. This test is conducted in the doctor's office to determine whether or not there is a significant vascular problem causing your ED. The doctor will inject a medication into your penis to initiate an erection. If there is a positive response (normal rigidity that lasts at least 20 minutes), your doctor will conclude that the blood vessels in your penis are functioning adequately to respond to injectable medications. A negative response (weak or no rigidity) will mean that you might have a significant penile vascular problem, for example, a venous leakage. However, a negative response can also occur because of a high level of anxiety caused by the testing environment and the concern about needles.

Penile Duplex Doppler Ultrasound (PDDU). This test is conducted by your doctor (usually a urologist) in his or her office to identify if your ED is due to a vascular (blood vessel) problem in the penis. Your doctor will initiate an erection of your penis through an injection similar to the abovementioned intracavernosal injection test. Then he or she will scan the erect penis with an ultrasound probe to measure the blood flow in the cavernosal artery during the erection.

Cavernosometry. Using an injection test and a measuring device, your doctor will use this study to check the blood flow and pressure in your penis. This test is designed to detect any venous leak-

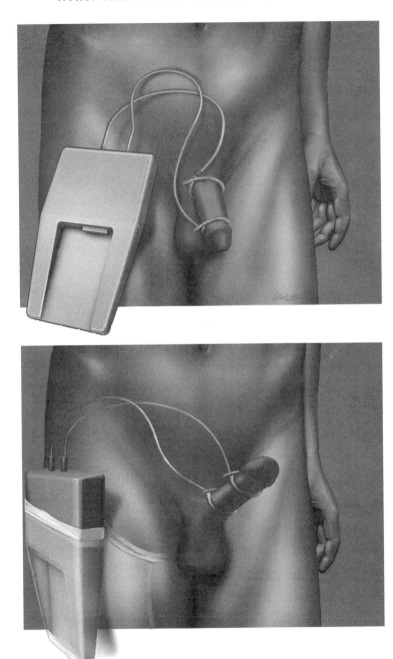

Figure 8. Recording of erections during sleep, or nocturnal penile tumescence and rigidity (NPTR). The two sensors of the portable RigiScan® device are connected to the penis prior to going to sleep. One sensor is placed at the base and the other at the tip of the penis.

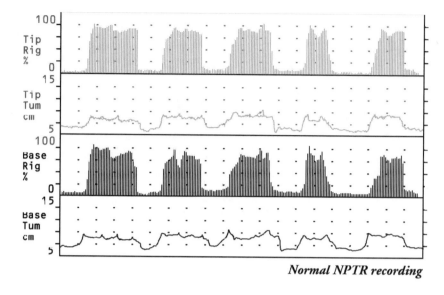

Normal NPTR recording

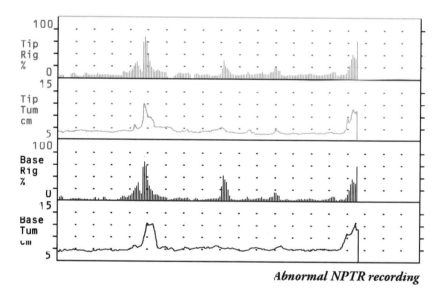

Abnormal NPTR recording

Figure 9. The RigiScan® device records data on the circumference and rigidity of the base and tip of the penis. The upper graph shows normal NPTR recording. In one night this man had five erections with excellent duration, increase in penile circumference, and rigidity, both at the base and the tip of the penis. The lower graph shows abnormal NPTR recording. In one night this man had two or three very short-lasting erections with minimal change in penile circumference and rigidity. The abnormal recording is both from the base and the tip of the penis.

age, which occurs when blood doesn't sufficiently remain in the penis, but leaks out.

Cavernosography. A dye is injected into the penis and then x-rays are taken to examine the venous leakage from the penis.

Penile Arteriography. A dye is injected into the arteries of the penis to detect any obstruction of the arteries.

Neurologic Testing

Biothesiometry. The various sensory capabilities of the penis are studied in comparison to other parts of the body, for example the fingers.

Bulbocavernosus Latency. This is a test to detect any nerve disease or injury by measuring the reflex-response time between stimulating the glans (head of the penis) and the contraction of the pelvic muscles.

Cavernosal EMG. This test records the electrical activity of the muscle cells of the erectile tissue of the penis.

Somatosensory Evoked Potential. This test measures the ability of the nerves to conduct sensation from a peripheral organ (the leg or the penis) to the spinal cord or the brain.

Endocrinologic Testing

Advanced Hormonal Tests. These blood tests check the hormones of the pituitary gland, including luteinizing hormone (LH), prolactin, and thyroid hormones, in addition to total and free testosterone.

MRI of the Brain. An image taken of the pituitary gland in the brain can rule out the possibility of the presence of a rare tumor.

Thyroid Function Studies. This blood test can check the function of the thyroid gland.

Once your doctor has adequate information to determine the nature of your problem, he or she will recommend the best treatment for you. However, not all men respond to the very first treatment option, so be sure to stay in touch with your doctor if you are not completely satisfied with the treatment results. A simple change in dosage or reinstruction about the use of medication can be all that is needed for success. There are many options for treatment (see Chapter V). If the first option doesn't live up to your expectations, consult your doctor and try something else. Don't give up trying and don't give up hope. There are new treatments and drugs coming on the market that will help expand your options to restore your sexual well-being.

THE PROCESS OF CARE

In December 1997 I participated in a conference with experts from different specialties to produce guidelines for the diagnosis and treatment of ED. These guidelines, called the Process of Care, were communicated to many doctors in the process of their continuing medical education and therefore formed the basis for the modern stepwise approach to the management of ED. Table 1 explains the steps in detail.

QUESTIONS MY PATIENTS ASK

Q: My wife and I have been arguing a lot lately and now I seem to have problems with getting an erection when I'm with her. Should I go and find another partner to test this out and see if I can really perform?

A: No. You should not be unfaithful and "experiment" with another partner. This can be dangerous to your health for several reasons and can also damage your emotional well-being. It would be much wiser for you to go and see your doctor. He or she can test your erection ability or lack thereof. Your doctor can also advise you on how to strengthen your relationship with your wife or direct you to a counselor. In short: "Don't check out your potency with a random partner."

TABLE 1

Process of Care Chart
for the Diagnosis and Treatment of ED

PROCESS	ACTION	OUTCOME
Process 1 Identification/Evaluation of ED	• Sexual, medical, and psychosocial history • Physical exam • Lab tests	• ED diagnosis confirmed. • Additional testing and/or referral if needed.
Process 2 Patient/Partner Assessment and Education	• Review of findings • Patient and partner education • Assessment of need for referral to specialist	• Identification of patient and partner needs and preferences. • Referral, if indicated and desired by patient.
Process 3 Modification of Reversible Causes	• Lifestyle modification • Discontinue or substitute medication • Hormonal replacement	• ED resolution with follow-up and reassessment. *or* • ED continues.
Process 4 First-Line Therapy	• Oral medication • Vacuum constriction device • Couples/sexual therapy	• ED resolution with follow-up and reassessment. *or* • ED continues.
Process 5 Second-Line Therapy	• Intraurethral therapy • Injection therapy	• ED resolution with follow-up and reassessment. *or* • ED continues.
Process 6 Third-Line Therapy	• Penile implant • Corrective surgery	• ED resolution with follow-up and reassessment.

With permission: *The Process of Care Model: Evaluation and Treatment of ED,* University of Medicine and Dentistry of New Jersey, Robert Wood Johnson Medical School, 1998.

Q: My wife does not want to come with me to the doctor. Is it necessary that she come with me for the evaluation and treatment of ED?

A: For the first visit, the most important thing is to start the process of evaluation and treatment, either alone or with your wife or partner. I usually recommend that the partner attend the second and/or subsequent visits. Sex is a joint project. Getting your partner involved will help you and her.

Q: Why does the diagnostic evaluation of ED involve so many questions?

A: The causes or risk factors for ED include many items that may not be mutually exclusive. Many patients have a combination of physical and psychological causes. Patients vary in their age, physical, psychological, and emotional status as well as their goals and concerns. In order to be able to help you effectively, your doctor needs to know about a wide range of aspects related to your health. This is an opportunity for you to have a comprehensive review of your general health in addition to your sexual health and ED.

Q: Should I tell the doctor about my personal sexual practices or about my alcohol and drug abuse?

A: Absolutely. Your relationship with your doctor is highly confidential. It is to the benefit of your health that your doctor knows about all your health issues and problems. This will enable your doctor to devise the appropriate treatment plan for you.

Q: Does my health insurance cover my visit to the doctor for the evaluation and treatment of ED?

A: Most insurance plans do. Check your insurance policy or call the insurance patient information number.

V

How to Treat ED

There are a variety of options for treating your ED. But you can't ignore it, or handle it all by yourself. ED is a progressive condition—it can only get worse, not better, without treatment. The best way to treat ED is with knowledge and open communication—with yourself, your partner, and with your doctor.

Knowledge is the key factor in treating ED. The more you know, the better you'll be equipped to know what works and what is just hype from illegitimate companies who make unsubstantiated promises that will only empty your wallet. You also need knowledge so you have the ability to describe your problem to your doctor, thus making it easier for the doctor or the team of healthcare professionals to develop a strategy of treatment that is just right for you and your partner.

Communication is another key to effectively treat ED. Ongoing dialogue with your partner and your doctor is critical to finding a treatment that is comfortable and effective. Your first treatment choice may not be effective or meet your expectations. Here's where you need to communicate with your doctor to make some adjustments. An open, honest and continuous dialogue will help in resolving your problem.

You'll need to carefully consider your options for treatment. Your doctor will certainly play a critical role in this, but if you are aware of the options, their effectiveness, side effects (complications), and costs, together with your partner and your doctor you can wisely choose the very best treatment—one that will not only be effective but will also restore satisfaction to your sex life.

The ideal therapy is:

- Simple to use
- Noninvasive (doesn't require surgery or an incision)
- Painless
- High success rate
- Brings your sex life closest to naturalness and spontaneity
- Few minor short-lasting side effects
- Affordable
- Satisfactory to your individual needs
- Satisfactory to you and your partner as a couple

As you read about these treatments before visiting your doctor, or as a review after your time together, keep the above criteria in mind.

In deciding on the method of treatment that is best for you, your doctor will take into consideration these factors: ease and convenience, cost, and degree of invasiveness. In most cases, he or she will start out with recommendations to fix or adjust the easy stuff (lifestyle adjustments) and move on to more advanced treatments. He or she will also take into consideration your personal desires and your level of determination for treatment. Just remember, no matter what kind of treatment you prefer, you need professional guidance and expertise.

YOU, ED, AND THE INTERNET

The Internet is a valuable source of information, but could never be a "virtual doctor." Nothing can replace the direct doctor–patient dialogue and interaction, or a physical exam. The quantity of information on the Net can sometimes be overwhelming, resulting in information overload, total confusion, and misunderstanding. The quality of information on the Net also varies tremendously from source to source. Some sources are merely

(Continued)

advertisements, preying on your insecurities and embarrassment to make you pay for worthless treatments. Others contain some reliable facts and some half-truths or unsubstantiated facts. Your doctor is your most reliable and professional source for information. Self-diagnosis is dangerous for any disease—including ED. Only the dialogue with your doctor can help you select the correct and beneficial information, diagnosis and treatment.

THINGS TO DO TO TREAT ED

- Call your doctor.
- Exercise.
- Pick up the phone (call your doctor).
- Stop smoking.
- Talk to your doctor.
- Educate yourself about ED.
- Call your doctor.
- Talk to your partner.
- Cut back on alcohol.
- Call your doctor.

LIFESTYLE ADJUSTMENTS

There are a few things you can do on your own to treat ED that have to do with your lifestyle. Only you can make adjustments and changes to how you live and conduct your life. Your doctor will ask you or remind you of these things, so start making some changes even before you see your doctor. Lifestyle changes alone may not completely cure ED, but they will definitely improve your general health and may improve your sexual situation.

Alcohol

Start keeping track of how much alcohol you *really* consume. Be honest with yourself. Does your glass of wine with dinner turn into three or four? Does an evening of relaxing after a hard day at work include two or three or more mixed drinks? Does the weekend out with friends include several cocktails before dinner, a few bottles of wine with dinner, and a nightcap or two?

According to some studies, consuming more than 600 ml of alcohol per week can be a risk factor for ED. One glass of wine is approximately 250 ml (one cup or 8 ounces): so if you have one glass of wine per night, every night of the week, you are consuming 1750 ml of alcohol per week (more than double the benchmark quantity).

Alcohol has both immediate and long-term effects on sexual

Macduff

What three things does drink especially provoke?

Porter

Marry, sir, nose-painting, sleep, and
urine. Lechery, sir, it provokes, and unprovokes;
it provokes the desire, but it takes
away the performance: therefore, much drink
may be said to be an equivocator with lechery:
it makes him, and it mars him; it sets
him on, and it takes him off; it persuades him,
and disheartens him; makes him stand to, and
not stand to; in conclusion, equivocates him
in a sleep, and, giving him the lie, leaves him.

—Shakespeare, *Macbeth*, Act 2, Scene 3, Porter answering Macduff function. The immediate effect is that it acts as a sedative, causing a weaker erection and decreasing the ability to have sex. Although many men think it increases their sex drive, it doesn't; it just diminishes inhibitions. Prolonged and excessive use of alcohol can damage the nerves through a condition called neuropathy.

Nicotine

If you are a cigarette smoker, you are twice as likely to experience ED. You already know that smoking is bad for your general health, potentially leading to lung cancer, heart disease, etc. Erectile dysfunction is another good reason to stop smoking.

Recreational Drugs

The use of marijuana, heroin, cocaine, and methadone is a risk factor in ED. These drugs are toxic to the nervous system, and if you use them over a long period of time, you will experience nerve damage. You may see an improvement in your sexual function if you discontinue use. Ecstasy is a dangerous new illegal drug that is readily available since it is easy to make, comes in tablet form, and is inexpensive enough for use by college and high school students. This drug intoxicates the nervous system and over time damages the central nervous system, which plays a vital role in normal sexual function.

Sedentary Lifestyle and General Health

As you've heard a thousand times, your general, overall health is important to your well-being. Being overweight or short of breath from basic activity or leading an inactive lifestyle can affect you in many ways—one of them is your sexual ability. Believe it or not, a sedentary lifestyle (i.e., being a couch potato) is bad for your sex life. So get up and get some exercise: walk, ride a bike, swim, play tennis or golf, rake the leaves, or go skiing. Proper lifestyle adjustments will enhance any other treatment you undertake.

Diabetes Control

If you are diabetic, get your diabetes under good control. Although ED is associated with diabetes in general, some studies have shown that poorly controlled diabetes or complicated diabetes poses a higher risk of ED than well-controlled diabetes. Getting your diabetes under good control has other health benefits too.

REVERSIBLE CAUSES

Hormone Therapy

Although lack of testosterone alone is an infrequent cause of ED, there are occasions when hormone therapy may be effective. Your doctor will be able to evaluate your testosterone levels through blood tests to determine your serum testosterone levels. As men age, it is common for them to experience a decline in sex hormones. This condition, called andropause or ADAM (Androgen Decline in the Aging Male), is characterized by:

- Decreased sexual function and libido
- Changes in mood including increased depression and anger
- Decrease in lean body mass and increased fat
- Decreased body hair
- Decreased bone density

These changes are due to a decline in testosterone, the main androgen secreted by males. The pros and cons of testosterone replacement therapy for older men are still being debated. Testosterone therapy is ineffective if there are normal hormone levels. In men over age 40, it is dangerous and inappropriate for any doctor to prescribe hormone therapy without first checking the prostate gland.

Testosterone replacement therapy is given as a regular intramuscular injection (DEPO®-Testosterone) every 2 to 3 weeks or in the form of a skin patch (Androderm® or Testoderm® TTS) that you can apply daily to your back, stomach, thighs, or upper arms. Recently, the FDA approved a new form of testosterone replacement therapy: a gel (AndroGel®) that is highly effective and well tolerated by the skin. AndroGel® has become the leader in testosterone therapy because of its effectiveness, excellent tolerability, and ease of use. Men using testosterone replacement therapy have noticed improvements in their sex drive, sexual function, energy, and mood.

Medications

All kinds of prescription drugs and over-the-counter medications can have a side effect of causing ED. Everything from cold and allergy medicines to medications for heart disease, high blood pressure, and ulcers can effect your sexual function.

If you suspect that your cold remedy or allergy medicine is causing your problem, be reassured that your condition is only temporary. You can either discontinue the use of the drug, switch to a different medication (ask your pharmacist which he or she would recommend), or wait till your cold is gone or hay fever season is over. Your problem should then be gone and your normal sexual function will return. More serious illnesses requiring prescribed medications must be considered more carefully with the help of your doctor.

Diuretics and beta-blockers used to control high blood pressure can cause ED. If you have been taking a medication for high blood pressure or heart disease for some time and then are confronted with ED, your medication is probably not the problem. However, if your doctor changes your dosage or your medication for some reason and suddenly you have ED, you should discuss it with him or her and ask if there is a possible connection between the two. (See Chapter III, pages 41–43.)

Never stop taking a prescribed medication without consulting your doctor. Untreated high blood pressure can affect major organs—the brain, eyes, heart, and kidneys—and do far more damage than causing ED. Your doctor may be able to change your medication or give you additional treatment for the ED. If you stop taking medication for your heart disease, you risk a lot more than just losing out on your sex life—you risk losing your life. One of your medications might be the cause of your ED, but only your doctor can determine that and advise you on the possible adjustment. Just as it is dangerous to self-medicate or overmedicate, it is dangerous to stop medication without professional advice.

FIRST-LINE THERAPY TREATMENTS

The multistep approach to the treatment of ED, recommended by the Process of Care panel and the 1st International Consultation on ED sponsored by the WHO, asks doctors to classify the various treatments for ED as first-, second-, or third-line therapies. Within each classification are several options to choose from. You, your doctor, and your partner should all discuss and understand the various options before choosing a treatment that you feel will work best for you. If one treatment within a classification does not work, your doctor will reevaluate your problem and recommend another dosage, an alternate medication, or another treatment. He or she will start with the simplest and easiest but effective treatment first, and then move on to the more aggressive therapies if it is needed.

Natural Treatments

Throughout time, man has sought ways to become more virile, to improve his sexual pleasure, and increase his performance. Myths and legends abound regarding natural substances from animals and plants, which when ingested, increase a man's virility. Spanish fly, rhinoceros horn, and oysters are just a few examples. Modern science has started pointing out that some natural substances might have some validity in improving our sex lives.

Unlike rhinoceros horn or oysters, natural chemicals found in ginkgo biloba and ginseng may have characteristics that affect certain factors critical for sexual performance.

There is an ongoing debate in the public and among physicians about the effectiveness of natural treatments (called neutraceuticals). Some physicians are cautiously encouraged by the initial testing results of some natural substances and are endorsing the use of ginkgo biloba, ginseng, L-arginine or combinations of these plus vitamins. The majority of physicians remain skeptical, citing that the tests have too few participating individuals, lack comparison with a placebo, have limited information on interaction with other drugs, and that test findings lack proof of safety and effectiveness. And yet many medical professionals, realizing that their patients yearn for an easy and natural way to treat their ED, continue to remain open-minded about prescribing neutraceuticals and eagerly review journal articles and test data pertaining to these natural remedies.

At this time, neutraceuticals are not recommended or condoned for use in patients with erectile dysfunction. That said, let's take a closer look at some of the natural substances available and what results are attributed to them. Natural remedies that are being examined as possible treatments for erectile dysfunction include:

Yohimbine is an alkaloid taken from the bark of the West African yohimbe tree. Some studies have shown that yohimbine increases blood flow to the penis, thus helping to attain an erection. Although yohimbine is not a recognized therapy for ED in most countries, some doctors do prescribe the drug for men with occasional erectile dysfunction where a physical cause is uncertain. Yohimbine hydrochloride is available by prescription. Dosage consists of taking 5.4 mg of the medication three times a day for two to three weeks to first know its effectiveness. Side effects include increased heart rate and blood pressure, anxiety, dizziness, headache, nausea, vomiting, and skin flushing.

The American Urological Association (AUA) has stated their

concern about the effectiveness of yohimbine for erectile dysfunction in men with physical causes of the problem. The AUA guidelines on the treatment of organic ED state that yohimbine is not much more effective than a placebo, though there may be mild effectiveness in men with psychological causes of ED. Some doctors believe that yohimbine is effective in selective patients. A study published in the February 1998 issue of *The Journal of Urology* stated that yohimbine is clinically slightly more effective than a placebo, regardless of the cause of the ED.

Ginkgo biloba is another medicinal herb that is said to help men with ED. Extract from the ginkgo leaf improves blood flow, particularly in the brain. In Europe ginkgo is widely prescribed for elderly patients with general problems of aging. Studies have shown that ginkgo also improves the blood flow to the penis and might be slightly effective in treating ED caused by the effects of diabetes. In the laboratory, ginkgo biloba extract was shown to produce relaxation of the penile erectile tissue, thus increasing circulation and blood flow to the penis, which *may* improve erectile function. In a most recent study, dosage was given of 40 to 60 mg twice daily showing some effectiveness. Side effects included stomach and intestinal upset, headache, allergic skin reactions, and the possibility of increased bruising.

L-arginine has been studied for the treatment of ED in several small studies. This natural substance may facilitate erection by relaxing the penile and vascular smooth muscle. Several clinical studies have reported only limited success using a wide variety of doses. It is obvious that more extensive studies are required to confirm the effectiveness and most appropriate use of this therapy.

Ginsenoside, the active ingredient extracted from ginseng, has been shown in lab tests to release increased levels of NO which induces relaxation of the corpus cavernosum, thus facilitating erection. In a recent study, ginsenoside was shown to be effective in patients with psychogenic ED, although none of the patients reported complete resolution of their ED.

ArginMax™ a dietary supplement consisting of L-arginine, ginkgo biloba, American and Korean ginseng, vitamins A, C, E, and B complex, and selenium and zinc, was recently evaluated in a small study of individuals experiencing mild to moderate ED. The results after four weeks of treatment showed some success with no significant side effects.

Chinese herbal mixture has been shown in the laboratory to improve erectile function in experimental animals that developed ED with a high cholesterol diet. Further studies are underway.

Natural remedies for ED have been around for centuries, but with the arrival of the miracle drug Viagra® (more on that later), the little blue pill that gives a simple solution to a complex medical problem, there has been an outpouring of bogus, "natural" medications that promise the same results as Viagra® but without a prescription. The manufacturers of these products tote their wares on the Internet, through mass ad mailings to AARP members, and on late-night TV, playing off the embarrassment, naiveté, wishful thinking, and desperation of men too proud or scared to consult their doctor. Most experts, including the Federal Trade Commission (FTC) agree that *most* "all-natural" or herbal products are not effective because there is no clinical proof of their effectiveness. If the promises sound almost too good to be true, they probably are. Don't pick up the phone, don't call today, don't reveal your credit card number to anyone who makes promises about an easy and natural fix for your erectile dysfunction. Do pick up the phone and call today—your internist, your urologist, or your primary care physician. Your doctor can evaluate your problem and counsel you in the very best method of treatment that has some clinical proof of its effectiveness. Your physician may very well be one who endorses the use of natural treatments and is eager and willing to guide you to the best neutraceuticals to remedy your problem. But you need a professional diagnosis before beginning any treatment, natural or otherwise.

FRAUD OR REAL?

With so many bogus over-the-counter treatments for ED available, the Federal Trade Commission (FTC) and sexual dysfunction experts offer these tips to consumers to evaluate treatment claims:

- *If the product is advertised as effective for treating impotence, and no physician's prescription is necessary, forget it. It probably won't work.*
- *If the product is advertised as a "breakthrough" in treating impotence, check with your doctor to see if it is legitimate.*
- *If the product claims to be promoted by a "medical organization" call your physician to check the credentials. Phony clinics and sham institutes are touting bogus cures for impotence.*
- *If the product claims to be scientifically proven to reverse impotence, check it out with your doctor. Some claims that "clinical studies" prove a product works are false; generally, high success rates should raise suspicions.*
- *If the product being pitched to cure impotence is herbal or all natural, be cautious. To date, no herb or all-natural substance has been shown to be 100 percent effective in the treatment of impotence.*

Note: If you suspect that a product for treating impotence is fraudulent, you may file a complaint with the FTC at its Web site, www.ftc.gov, or by writing to the FTC Consumer Response Center at CRC, Washington, D.C. 20580, or calling 202-FTC-HELP.

Natural products are widely used even though many doctors are concerned that insufficient testing has been conducted to verify the safety and effectiveness of these treatments. Nevertheless, interest in additional research and development of natural products for treating ED remains very high. Our New York Center of Human Sexuality and the Holistic Urology Center continue to research and evaluate new treatments and to provide counseling to patients with ED who ask about natural remedies.

Oral Medications

Since oral medications are a convenient, easy, and noninvasive treatment, "popping a pill" is the most popular treatment within the first-line therapy classification. And since the arrival of *Viagra*® (sildenafil citrate), in 1998, everyone with ED believes it to be the miracle treatment. Perhaps it is. However, the miracle may be that the introduction and exposure of Viagra® has encouraged men to start discussing and seeking treatment for their sexual problem. The entry of this little blue pill into the marketplace, and its overwhelming success, has made it the catalyst that destroyed the shroud of secrecy surrounding sexual problems. Sex is now talked about more openly, not only in private, among friends and family, but in the public sphere: on television, in the movies, and on the Internet. When an elected official such as former Senator Bob Dole can feel comfortable discussing his sexual ailment by endorsing Viagra®, the male population in general feels empowered to also share their sexual situation.

The discovery of Viagra® was a modern breakthrough that revolutionized the treatment of erectile dysfunction. The researchers of the drug company, Pfizer, first stumbled onto the medication around 1992 while conducting research for the treatment of angina (chest pain caused by blocked blood vessels in the heart). These scientists were thinking about abandoning the angina project when they realized that some patients were reporting erections as a side effect of the medication they were being given. Pfizer knew immediately that it had accidentally hit gold— a drug that could stimulate blood vessels in the penis, and yet have little effect on the rest of the body.

After much controversy, testing, and waiting, the U.S. Food and Drug Administration (FDA) approved sildenafil citrate for the treatment of erectile dysfunction in March 1998. This date will always be remembered as the first time an oral drug was approved to fight erectile dysfunction—and with incredible success!

Knowing the chemistry of what causes an erection will help you understand how Viagra® works in the body. After investigating the drug, researchers concluded that Viagra® blocks or hinders PDE-5 action, so that the chemical cGMP continues its role in keeping the penis rigid. Remember that cGMP is the chemical produced during arousal in response to stimulation. With PDE-5 hindered, the faucet is left open, so to speak. The blood vessels remain broadened and engorged within the penis, the erection is more easily maintained, and the chances of an erection ending prematurely are significantly reduced (see Figure 10). Now we understand that Viagra® belongs to the class of medications called "PDE-5 inhibitors." Since Viagra® was discovered, other PDE-5 inhibitors have entered the field of research and development. Such medications include Cialis™ and Vardenafil, which are in the process of evaluation by the FDA as this book goes to press.

Researchers made another discovery while studying Viagra® and the other PDE-5 inhibitors Cialis™ and Vardenafil: they work so well because they very specific medications. In other words, Viagra®, Cialis™, Vardenafil, and other future PDE-5 inhibitors have a selective effect on the physiology of the penis but have little or limited side effects on the rest of the body. It was this specific selectivity feature that led the researchers to abandon the Viagra® angina project. They learned that Viagra® was incapable of significantly dilating the blood vessels of the heart, and therefore, was not a successful treatment for angina. It was this very factor that made Viagra® such an effective oral medicine for erectile dysfunction. Luck often plays a significant part in the discovery of new drugs, and the story of Viagra® is a testament to this fact. The discovery of PDE-5 inhibitors such as Viagra®, is nothing short of remarkable!

Viagra® is not a cure-all treatment, but it is a highly effective and very safe medication. It has been shown to help in the treatment of about 70% of all erectile dysfunction patients. Among the side effects that have been documented, about 16% of users report headaches, 10% flushing (redness of the face), 7% upset stomach, 4% nasal congestion (stuffy nose), and approximately 3% complain of altered vision. These side effects are usually mild

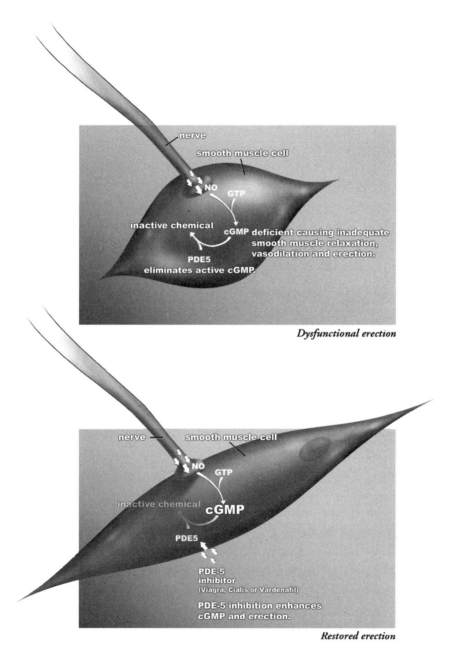

Dysfunctional erection

Restored erection

Figure 10. How PDE-5 inhibitors (Viagra®, Cialis™, or Vardenafil) work. PDE-5 inhibitors enhance erection by stopping the enzyme PDE-5 in the penis from breaking down cGMP, which
is the natural substance (neurotransmitter) causing erection. cGMP is produced in the penis
in response to production of nitric oxide (NO) with sexual stimulation.

to moderate and rarely severe. They last only a few hours. There are no long-term side effects to Viagra®.

Few patients need to stop using Viagra® or any of the other oral medications as a result of side effects. However, patients using medications containing nitrates must avoid Viagra® like the plague. Mixing nitrates and Viagra® can cause blood pressure to plummet, possibly causing a heart attack, a stroke, or even death! Viagra® is strictly contraindicated in patients using nitrates in any shape, form, dose, or frequency.

The effect of Viagra® lasts up to 4 hours after you take it. This does not mean that you would have a continuous erection for 4 hours. Viagra® only works when a man is sexually stimulated. If sexual stimulation stops, so does the erection. Viagra® doesn't increase your sex drive, change fertility, or increase sexual prowess. It doesn't cure ED: one pill or dose equals a period of about 4 hours of being ready for sex. During this period you may have more than one erection and more than one sexual encounter. But you may only take Viagra® once a day. Viagra® takes time to work but with stimulation it will help you attain an erection in approximately 30 to 60 minutes.

• If you are taking nitrate-containing medications (usually prescribed for coronary heart disease or angina), do not use Viagra® or other PDE-5 inhibitors such as Cialis™ and Vardenafil. The combination of nitrates and Viagra® or other PDE-5 inhibitors might cause a dangerous and life-threatening drop in blood pressure.

• Viagra®, Cialis™, and Vardenafil require sexual stimulation to work and to continue working. When sexual stimulation stops, a Viagra®-induced erection stops.

• Although very rare with Viagra® and the other oral medications, if you experience an erection lasting longer than 4 hours, you should call your doctor or visit the closest emergency room immediately.

For most patients, Viagra® works the first or second time you take it. However, it may work better the third or fourth time. If Viagra® is not effective, keep trying it at least four times, at the maximum dose that your doctor prescribes for you, before declaring it as ineffective and moving on to the second-line therapy.

You need to take Viagra® on an empty stomach. Avoid eating a heavy, fatty meal and drinking too much alcohol before you ingest this medication. A steak dinner and two bottles of wine might delay or prevent the drug from being effective. However Viagra® is safe to take with aspirin, Coumadin®, antacids, or a small amount of alcohol, since there is no harmful interaction.

Never use Viagra® without a prescription from your doctor after a complete medical evaluation. Don't take a friend's prescription or order pills over the Internet or buy it on the street corner. Your doctor is the only one who can determine what dosage is right for you to treat your problem. Viagra® comes in three strengths: 25, 50, and 100 mg tablets. Most of the time 50 mg is prescribed initially, but if that dose is not effective, let your doctor know so he or she can increase the dose. For patients over 65, those who have severe liver and kidney disease, or those taking

---

DO'S AND DON'TS FOR TAKING VIAGRA®

Do's

• *Do take Viagra® on an empty stomach.*

• *Do give Viagra® time to work (30 to 60 minutes).*

• *Do participate in sexual stimulation after taking Viagra®.*

• *Do visit your doctor if your dosage isn't effective.*

Don'ts

• *Don't take Viagra® with a medication containing nitrates.*

• *Don't eat a fatty meal before taking Viagra®.*

• *Don't take more than one pill per day.*

• *Don't buy Viagra® over the Internet or on the street corner.*

• *Don't give a "sample" of your Viagra® to a friend.*

medications like cimetidine (Tagamet®), erythromycin, ketocona-zole, or protease inhibitors (medications for treating the AIDS virus HIV), your doctor may start at the lower dose of 25 mg.

You should try Viagra® a minimum of four times, or a maximum of eight times, before you and your doctor make a judgment as to whether or not it is working.

New Treatments Are on the Way

Soon Viagra® will no longer be the only oral medication available for treating ED. Several others are currently being tested, and might be approved soon.

Cialis™ (tadalafil or IC_{351}) is a new oral PDE-5 inhibitor, enhancing erectile function by blocking the enzyme PDE-5 (see Figure 10). Clinical tests have proven that Cialis™ is effective in treating erectile dysfunction of various causes, resulting in significant patient satisfaction. Cialis™ is a long-acting medication and therefore has been proven to be effective for up to 24 hours. Dosages of up to 25 mg were very well tolerated by participants in the clinical studies with only minor side effects of headache, back pain, and indigestion. Because of its long-acting feature, Cialis™

FACTS ABOUT PDE-5 INHIBITORS: VIAGRA®, CIALIS™ AND VARDENAFIL

• *PDE-5 inhibitors can be prescribed by your primary care physician or a specialist.*

• *Before Viagra®, fewer than 1 in 20 men (i.e., 5%) with ED sought help.*

• *Currently 1 in 4 men (i.e., 25%) with ED seek help.*

• *PDE-5 inhibitors are not habit-forming.*

• *Patients do not develop a tolerance to PDE-5 inhibitors.*

• *PDE-5 inhibitors do not cure ED, they are a treatment for ED.*

• *Treatments for ED do not protect you or your partner from getting sexually transmitted diseases, including HIV (the virus that causes AIDS). Continue to practice safe sex.*

• *Viagra®, Cialis™, and Vardenafil are not hormones or an aphrodisiac.*

is expected to provide men with ED an option of treatment with an opportunity to restore spontaneity to sexual function and remove the annoying element of "planning for sex." Similar to Viagra®, this medication is contraindicated with any type of nitrates. The New Drug Application (NDA) for Cialis™ was submitted to the FDA in June 2001. It may be approved and marketed in 2002.

Vardenafil is another oral PDE-5 inhibitor that enhances erections by increasing smooth muscle relaxation and vasodilation (see Figure 10). This drug is highly selective and potent in inhibiting PDE-5, which is present primarily in the erectile tissue of the penis. This drug has been tested in doses of 5, 10, 20, or 40 mg. Vardenafil has proven to be safe, well tolerated (few side effects), and effective in producing erections. In laboratory tests, it is more potent than Viagra®, so a lesser dosage is necessary to achieve the same results. About 70 percent of patients using Vardenafil achieved erections. The drug is taken once a day as needed. Mild headache is the most significant side effect. Vardenafil, like Viagra®, may not be taken with a medication containing nitrates. The New Drug Application for Vardenafil (NDA) was submitted to the FDA in September 2001 and is expected to be approved and marketed in 2002.

Again, these three medications—Viagra®, Cialis™, and Vardenafil—all enhance erections by inhibiting PDE-5, thereby enhancing smooth muscle relaxation, vasodilation, and erection in response to sexual stimulation.

Sublingual apomorphine (Uprima® or Ixense®) is absorbed rapidly via the mouth. It reaches the erection centers in the central nervous system to produce an erection (see Figure 11). It is effective in 10 to 25 minutes when enhanced with sexual arousal and stimulation and can be taken more than once per day at a minimum interval of 8 hours.

ED patients in several studies have reported erections firm enough for intercourse 40 to 60 percent of the time. Unlike Viagra®, Uprima® can be taken by patients who are also taking nitrates.

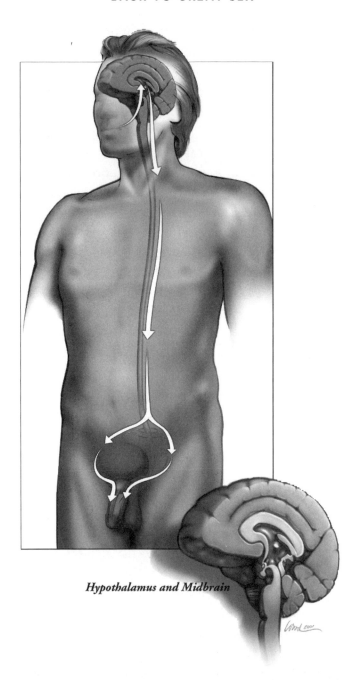

Hypothalamus and Midbrain

Figure 11. How sublingual apomorphine (Uprima® or Ixense®) works. It activates the erection centers in the brain, which in turn send signals down the spinal cord and subsequently to the penis to enhance erection in response to sexual stimulation.

The most common side effect is nausea, which is generally mild and tends to diminish with repeated doses. Other side effects include headache, sweating, dizziness, sleepiness, and yawning. A few men (0.3% at the recommended dose) have had brief episodes of fainting (syncope), generally preceded by sweating, nausea, and dizziness. All recovered and none who continued taking Uprima® fainted again. Because of the risk of fainting, however, it is advisable not to drive or perform hazardous tasks for 2 hours after taking Uprima®.

In April 2000, a committee of the FDA recommended that sublingual apomorphine (Uprima® or Ixense®) in doses of 2, 3, and 4 mg be approved for the treatment of erectile dysfunction. However, the pharmaceutical manufacturer withdrew the application at the end of June 2000 to do more testing regarding Uprima®'s safety. In January 2001, Uprima® was approved in the European Union countries at doses of 2 mg and 3 mg. Since the approval status of Uprima® in the United States could change at any time, check with your doctor for the latest news. Or check the website www.ClinicalTrials.gov to see if this drug is in final testing.

Phentolamine (Vasomax®). A 40 mg oral dose has been shown to be moderately effective, with an erection occurring in as little as 20 minutes. Clinical tests have shown that it is effective in 37 to 45 percent of patients with mild ED. Side effects include headache, nasal stuffiness, and facial flushing in less than 10 percent of the participants. It is currently available in Mexico and Brazil (under the brand name of Vasomax®) but it is not available in the United States owing to safety reasons. Clinical testing of this drug in the U.S. has stopped, also for safety reasons. It is uncertain at this time whether further testing and application for approval by the FDA for human use will continue.

Vacuum Erection Therapy
Although oral medication is the preferred method of treatment by both doctors and patients, there are times when that

treatment is not effective, or is incompatible with other medications already being taken, such as nitrates. In such cases your doctor may recommend that you try alternate treatments that have been used for several decades and have proven to be very effective.

A vacuum constriction device (VCD) draws blood into the penis, causing an erection. The system consists of a plastic cylinder, a vacuum pump, a connecting tube, and constriction bands or rings. The plastic cylinder is placed over the penis. The battery-operated or manual pump draws the air out of the cylinder, creating a vacuum. The negative pressure in the cylinder forces blood to engorge the penis and create an erection. The constriction band (an elastic ring) is then slipped around the base of the penis to maintain the erection by keeping the blood in the penis (see Figure 12).

How the Vacuum Device Works

1. After lubricating your penis, especially at the base, place it inside the cylinder. Activate the pump to produce a vacuum inside the cylinder to pull blood into the penis.
2. Slip the constrictive ring off the cylinder, onto the base of your penis. Remove the cylinder. Now you can safely and easily keep the erection for up to 30 minutes, using only the constrictive ring.
3. To end the erection, remove the ring and your penis will return to its soft state.

The time it takes to achieve an erection is generally between 2 to 2.5 minutes; however, the constriction ring cannot be left in place for more than 30 minutes at a time. Vacuum devices available with a prescription are well tried and tested and are approved by the FDA. This treatment is effective and safe. It does not introduce another drug into the body, it can be used whenever and as often as desired, and it has a relatively low cost. Although it is listed as a first-line therapy, it can be used at any step in your process of achieving full sexual function. Its popularity, however, is limited, mainly because the vacuum constriction device is a

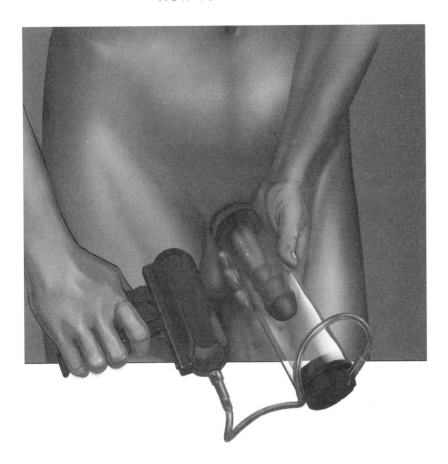

Figure 12. How a vacuum constriction device works. After lubricating the penis, especially at the base, it is placed inside the cylinder. The pump is activated to produce a vacuum inside the cylinder to pull blood into the penis. The vacuum will allow you to create a near-natural erection within a few minutes. The constrictive ring is moved off the cylinder onto the base of the penis. The cylinder is removed and sexual activity begins. To end the erection, the ring is removed and the penis returns to its soft state.

rather large mechanical object that many couples consider a major, unromantic interruption in their lovemaking. Satisfaction with the results varies greatly: as few as 27 percent to as high as 69 percent participants in some studies were satisfied. Men and their partners were dissatisfied with this method for the following reasons: inability to maintain a full erection, bruising or pain in the

penis, inconvenience or awkwardness of the device, problem ejaculating, cooling and discoloration of the penis. Most vacuum constriction devices come with an instructional videotape and a
booklet to ensure your success in using the device.

Venous Flow Controllers (VFCs)

In some men, ED is due to the inability to store trapped
blood in the penis, necessary to sustain an erection. The blood
"leaks out" through the veins, thus the name "venous leakage."
VFCs are rubber or plastic rings, made with a certain amount of
tension and flexibility, that are placed at the base of the penis in
order to prevent the blood from exiting the erect penis too
quickly. VFCs are available with a prescription but have not
proven to be very effective. Patients complain about their penis
getting numb owing to too-tight constriction.

> *Vacuum devices are the oldest form of treatment for ED. In 1694 J. van
> Musschenbrack in Leiden, Netherlands, described experiments with vac-
> uum air pumps. In 1874 an American, John King, used the vacuum device
> in a clinical setting. Dr. Otto Lederer in 1917 added compression to the de-
> vice. In an attempt to improve his own sexual performance, Gedding
> Osbon in 1960 developed a device, which became commercially available
> in 1975, but was not marketed until 1982. Osbon's device is now known as
> ErecAid®, currently marketed by Timm Medical.*

Counseling and Sex Therapy

Another option in the first-line therapy category is counseling and/or sex therapy. Although it is frequently considered a first-
choice option, counseling and sex therapy will also be beneficial
with any second- or even third-line therapies. At any time if a psychological or relationship issue comes up, sex therapy can always
be helpful. Individual counseling may be necessary to help you address any anger, low self-esteem, depression, or anxiety you're

feeling as a result of your ED. If you haven't sought help for your ED problem for many years, there may be several unresolved issues that you need to express, share, acknowledge, and resolve with the help of a professional.

A *professional counselor* will be able to help you deal with your personal emotional problems: depression, anger, need for control, aggression, self-esteem, self-image, and relationships in general. A *marriage counselor,* on the other hand, will address the emotional needs within your marital relationship and help you find ways to improve the harmony in your marriage as well as your sexual relationship as a couple.

A *sex therapist* is a trained professional who knows how to listen nonjudgmentally and to talk about your emotional and physical sexual issues. He or she can address any issues you are having with your partner regarding sex: motivation, physical readiness, knowledge in techniques, and resuming sex after ED (no matter what the reason). They also can coach you to change any ineffective sexual behaviors or any negative sexual attitudes and poor self-image. Sex therapy usually consists of six to fourteen visits, meeting weekly or biweekly. Brief therapy of two to eight sessions may be needed for those who are struggling with their perception that a certain ED treatment is unnatural or an unacceptable way to satisfy their sexual desires.

The key to effective and short-term therapy is communication. Being open and honest and providing detailed information about your sexual practices and problems will assist your therapist in helping you overcome your problems and return to a healthy sex life. Holding back information will only hinder your own progress and may even hinder the effectiveness of any other ED treatment you are simultaneously using.

Through discussion and openness, a sex therapist will begin to understand your needs and your partner's needs and desires. He or she will then assign some structured erotic exercises for you to practice alone or with your partner privately at home. These experiences will help you have a positive sexual experience that will restore you to sexual health and sexual harmony in your relationship.

During the 1990s sex therapy was not promoted for treatment of ED due to the advances in medical and surgical approaches; however, since the arrival of oral medications such as Viagra® in 1998, sex therapy is now playing a significant role in improving the overall effectiveness and extended satisfaction of patients with the prescribed treatment. Medications can easily restore an erection for the physical side of sex, but in many cases, there are other sexual issues that only sex therapy or counseling can address. If these other issues are not resolved, Viagra®, or any other medical treatments, may not be effective. In contrast, a combination of medical treatment and sex therapy will not only be more effective but will also shorten the time needed for therapy.

Sex therapy will help you:
- *Overcome a negative self-image*
- *Make your medical treatment more effective*
- *Learn how to effectively incorporate treatment into your life*
- *Restore spontaneity to your love life*
- *Resolve desire differences between you and your spouse*
- *Address some female partner issues*
- *Address issues of stress, fatigue, mood, anger, substance abuse, and relationship problems*
- *Improve techniques for sexual response, creating desire, excitement, orgasm, and resolution*
- *Adjust self-defeating sexual attitudes*
- *Motivate you to keep trying after experiencing treatment failure*

Sex therapy helps you understand that sex is more than an erection (even though a good one does help). An erection alone will not restore you to a satisfying sex life and a happy marriage. You also need to incorporate the power of intimacy, pleasure, and eroticism. If your doctor refers you to a sex therapist, don't resist.

Addressing your physical and emotional needs simultaneously will provide you with a strong, healthy, and lasting sex life.

SECOND-LINE THERAPY TREATMENTS

Your doctor will recommend a therapy from the second-line therapy treatments when and if oral medications are ineffective, or conflict with other medications you are taking, or if you and your partner have a preference for an alternate treatment. If your primary care physician does not deliver second- and third-line therapies for ED, you could or should request a referral to a urologist. Most primary care physicians do not utilize self-injection therapy and only urologists perform penile implant surgery.

Self-Injection Therapy

Self-injection therapy is the most effective and popular therapy of the second-line treatments. But I know what you're thinking. Just the thought of this treatment makes you cringe and react with an emphatic "No way!" But trust me, the anticipation is far worse than the event. For most men the sensation of the injection is no worse than pinching an earlobe. Many of my patients are pleasantly surprised after experiencing their first injection in my office. Many of them never feel the injection and ask, "Have you done it yet?" when I'm already finished.

Available since 1982, injection therapy hit the commercial market in 1995 and was touted as a major medical breakthrough. Up until the recent arrival of oral medication, injection therapy was the "gold standard" of treatment for ED. This treatment has proven to be highly effective and the results are very satisfying to most users and their partners.

Self-injection therapy involves injecting medication into the side of the shaft of the penis prior to sexual activity. The medication goes into the corpus cavernosum, where it relaxes the smooth

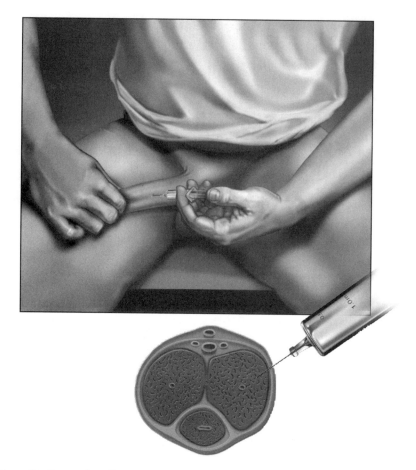

Figure 13. How penile self-injection is done. The penis is held from the head (the glans) and pulled straight on the thigh. The skin of the side of the shaft of the penis is cleaned with an alcohol swab. The needle is inserted at right angles into the side of the penis. The medication goes directly into one corpus cavenosum.

muscle cells, dilates the blood vessels and creates an erection within 5 to 20 minutes that is firm enough for intercourse (see Figure 13).

The most common, best studied, best documented, and only medication approved by the FDA for injection therapy is *prostaglandin E$_1$* (PGE$_1$), or *alprostadil.* Prostaglandin E$_1$ is a smooth muscle relaxant and vasodilator. It is available in two commercial forms: alprostadil sterile powder (Caverject®) and alprostadil-alfadex (Edex® in the United States and Viridal® in Europe). Erections usually occur within 5 to 20 minutes following injection. Since every person responds to the drug differently, your doctor will give you a "custom" dosage to ensure your erections last 45 to 60 minutes. The most practical dosage is 5 to 40 mcg. You should be aware that an injection-induced erection will last for a full 45 to 60 minutes. Even if you experience orgasm and ejaculation before the time is up, your erection will remain intact until the medication wears off. However, the orgasm and ejaculation remain pleasurable.

Testing has proven alprostadil to have a success rate of 73 to 94 percent. The main side effect is pain in the penis, not from the actual injection but from the medication itself. Some degree of pain occurs in approximately 30 percent of patients during the trial period and in approximately 15 percent of patients during long-term treatment. Long-term studies have shown that the use of prostaglandin E_1 injection therapy significantly improves the quality of life and satisfactory sexual intercourse for both the patient and his partner. Prostaglandin E_1 has proven to be extremely safe and have long-term effectiveness. Studies have shown that penile injection therapy with prostaglandin E_1 (either Caverject® or Edex®/Viridal®) is highly effective and satisfactory in patients who have failed to respond to Viagra®.

A recent development in the use of injection therapy is the introduction of Caverject Impulse® (in some countries it might be marketed under the name Caverject Dual Chamber®, Caverject Dual®). This new product has the same medication (alprostadil) as the original Caverject®. But alprostadil in powdered form is provided in a dual chamber with sterile water in the other chamber. The advantages of this new Caverject® include easier mixing of the powder and sterile water, easier setting of the dosage, and shorter time of preparation for injection.

Although prostaglandin E_1 is the most widely used drug for self-injection therapy, several other available drugs have been proven effective in the treatment of ED. The use of these drugs for the treatment of ED is not approved by the FDA and therefore their use is considered "off label." These drugs include papaverine and phentolamine in various mixtures.

Bimix is a mixture of two drugs—papaverine and phentolamine. Numerous reports have been published confirming that this combination is very effective and safe for injection therapy. Nineteen reports using this drug have shown that 72 percent of the patients achieved erections adequate for intercourse when using bimix. There was a low incidence of pain and relatively few adverse side effects.

Trimix is a combination of three drugs: papaverine, phentolamine, and PGE_1. A report on 210 patients treated with trimix showed that 81 percent of the patients achieved an adequate erection with a low incidence of adverse effects. Trimix has also been proven effective in patients who were not successful using bimix.

Bimix and trimix are not drugs available in and of themselves. They are combinations of two or three drugs that are available only as compounded medications—special mixtures prepared by a urologist or a compounding pharmacy that mixes this special formula through a prescription.

Should you and your urologist agree on your use of self-injection therapy, your urologist will carefully instruct you in the process of injecting yourself. You'll try the first few injections in the doctor's office to find out if you respond to the treatment, to determine if the dosage is effective or needs adjustment, and to train you in the technique of injecting yourself. Your urologist will start you on a small test dose and then increase the dose gradually until a satisfactory rigid erection lasting 45 to 60 minutes is achieved. The reason for the gradual dose increase is to prevent overdosage and prolonged erection, or *priapism*. You will probably practice in front of your urologist two or three different times to be sure you have successfully mastered the technique. Spending the time with your urologist and making the effort to learn the process are well worth it.

The following instructions for the use of Caverject® are simple and with practice will become routine.

1. Reconstitute the powder form of the drug and fill the syringe with medication.
2. Hold the penis from the head (the glans). Pull the penis tight and lay it on your thigh.
3. Wipe the skin of the side of the shaft of the penis with an alcohol swab.
4. Holding the needle and syringe at right angles to the penis, insert the needle into the side of the shaft of the penis. Avoid inserting the needle through the top or the bottom sides. Do not inject into the head.
5. Inject the medication directly into one corpus cavenosum, avoiding any veins on the surface.
6. Compress the injection site for 3 to 5 minutes.
7. Vary the location of the injection site with each use.

Some possible side effects that you should be aware of are pain, bleeding or bruising at the injection site, scarring (fibrosis), or prolonged erection (priapism). Although fibrosis occurs in less than 10 percent of patients, it is important to visit your urologist for checkups so he or she can examine the penis for the early signs of fibrosis. If the fibrosis is progressive, you will have to stop injection therapy.

Prolonged erections can be very painful and, if not treated, can cause damage to the penis. The blood that flows into the penis to create an erection becomes trapped, loses oxygen and nutrients due to lack of circulation, and turns toxic. This side effect is rare and completely avoidable by following dosage instructions and increasing the injection dosage gradually. Remember that any erection that continues uninterrupted for more than four hours turns from pleasure into an emergency! You must seek medical help immediately. Call your urologist or go to the emergency room of the hospital. A counteracting medication will be injected into the penis to end the prolonged erection. Injection therapy may be used once a day, two to three times a week. Advances in this treatment include special automatic injectors that are easy to use and visually appealing. Prior to 1998 and the introduction of oral medications, injection therapy was the standard treatment for ED, with 75 percent of men choosing this treatment. Even though there is now Viagra® and, in the future, other oral medications, some men cannot use these drugs or do not respond to them. Injection therapy continues to be safe and effective in treating ED, no matter what the cause. Many men find that they prefer the injections, even if given a choice, because they can count on the consistent and quick results.

Intraurethral Therapy

For men who are averse to injection therapy, there is another method of administering the drug alprostadil in the form of a soft pellet suppository inserted into the urethra (the urinary channel in the penis). The medication causes the blood vessels to relax, allowing the penis to fill with blood, resulting in an erection within 10 minutes. Most erections are not rigid but are adequate for intercourse and are maintained for 30 or 60 minutes. You can use this method more frequently than other ED treatments: twice in a 24-hour period.

The intraurethral therapy applicator is about an inch long and an eighth-inch wide. It is plastic and disposable. This method of treatment is referred to as MUSE® (Medicated Urethral System for Erection) and is relatively safe and somewhat effective, although not as effective as injection therapy. The range of men responding to MUSE® with an erection adequate for intercourse is about 43 percent.

The steps for administering MUSE® are as follows (see Figure 14):

1. Be sure to urinate before administering this medication.
2. Insert the applicator stem into the urethra.
3. Depress the applicator button.

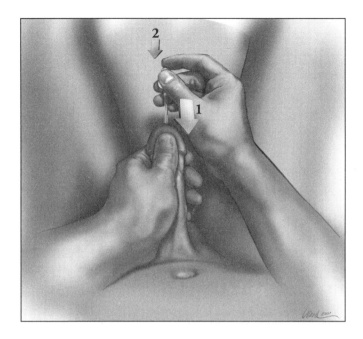

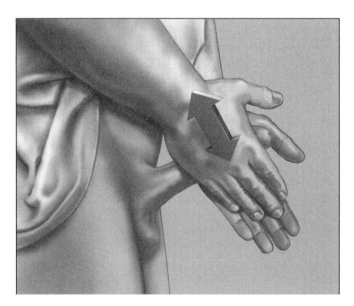

Figure 14. How intraurethral therapy (MUSE®) is used. The applicator stem is inserted into the urethra. Then the applicator button is depressed to deliver the medication. The applicator is removed after delivery of the medication. Subsequently, the penis is held upright and rolled between the hands to distribute the medication and improve absorption.

4. Remove the applicator.
5. Hold the penis upright and roll it between your hands
   for at least 10 seconds to distribute the drug and improve
   absorption.

Side effects from this treatment include penile or groin pain, low
blood pressure, burning sensation, or minor bleeding in the urethra. The medication, alprostadil, may irritate the vagina of your
partner, causing a slight burning or itching. You should not use this
therapy if your partner is pregnant or plans to become pregnant.

In studies comparing the effectiveness, safety, and patient's
preference of injection therapy with alprostadil (Caverject® or
Edex®/ Viridal®) with MUSE®, patients with ED found that injection therapy with Caverject® or Edex® was better at producing an
erection sufficient for sexual intercourse than MUSE®. Patient and
partner satisfaction was greater with Caverject® or Edex® and
more patients preferred this therapy, choosing to continue it after
the study. Since injection therapy has been proven to be more effective, better tolerated, and preferred by patients and their partners over intraurethral therapy, injection therapy may be your first
choice of treatment should you be unable to take oral medications.

> Caution: If you are using either intraurethral or MUSE® therapy or a topi-
> cal gel of prostaglandin E₁, do not let your partner give you oral sex. If your
> partner ingests this drug, your partner's throat could swell causing diffi-
> culty in breathing.

Topical Gels and Ointments

Topical therapy through gels and ointments applied to the
penis has a high appeal to many men and their partners; there are
no needles or mechanical devices to contend with. Even though
the variety of oral medications for treating erectile dysfunction

continues to grow, there is still a strong desire to create a gel or a cream that is effective, safe, and easy to apply.

Topical medications may have several advantages over other therapies. For example, gels:

- May work faster than oral medications.
- Are noninvasive.
- Do not cause scar tissue (fibrosis).
- Work directly on the penis—where it's needed—not on the entire body.

Although ointments and gels have the potential for being a good therapy, they are presently being studied in clinical trials and are not yet available for general use. The only drug presently being tested in gel form for application to the glans penis is prostaglandin E_1. Clinical trials are promising.

Prostaglandin E_1 (alprostadil) relaxes the smooth muscle of the corpora cavernosa in the penis. Various forms of alprostadil (injections, urethral suppositories, and gels) have been tested over the past 15 years for the treatment of ED. There have been a few studies with promising results that alprostadil in gel form helps in attaining an erection. Studies show that this drug, under the name of Topiglan, was effective in laboratory testing. Alprox-TD is another promising topical gel using alprostadil that is presently in clinical trials. Further studies, however, must be completed to substantiate these results as well as to consider the effects the drug has on the partner.

THIRD-LINE THERAPY TREATMENT

Penile Implants
The Rolls-Royce of all treatments is the penile implant. If you are looking for a permanent solution for your ED, want predictable and reliable outcome, almost instantaneous erections,

low risk, extremely satisfying results, and resumption of satisfying sex for you and your partner, then this procedure is for you.

Prior to the introduction of oral and self-injection therapies, penile implants were the most popular treatment for ED. Implants were introduced about 30 years ago, and were the first treatment for organic (physical) erectile dysfunction. Over the years, bio-medical engineering has vastly improved the implants. They continue to be an effective treatment for men desiring a permanent solution for their ED and for men who do not respond to oral or topical medications.

The greatest advantage of an implant is the final result. An inflatable implant yields a very natural, reliable, and available erection (there is no time lapse to achieve an erection). The results are truly wonderful, effective, and satisfying. Men who could no longer have intercourse owing to ineffective oral and/or topical treatments find that after implant surgery they can resume their sex life and be intimate whenever and as often as they choose. Over 90 percent of men and their partners are satisfied with the results of this treatment.

On the other hand, penile implant, the last resort for treating erectile dysfunction, is invasive (requires surgery), expensive, and associated with a few complications. This procedure cannot be reversed, and since surgery is required, you will need to carefully consider this option even after all other treatments have failed. The implant is carefully fitted inside your body and all the mechanical parts are hidden internally. Following implant surgery, all of your erections will require the use of the implant, so you must have it for life.

Some men have a few complaints after having an implant:

- Sensitivity is diminished after surgery.
- Their erection with the implant is not as long or as rigid as previously.
- They have difficulty inflating and deflating the implant.

- There is occasional spontaneous inflation.
- They have difficulty concealing a semirigid implant.
- They fail to reach orgasm.

These concerns and observations arise in a minority of those who have an implant. The majority of men and their partners are very satisfied.

Types of Implants

There are two types of implants: malleable (bendable) or semirigid rods, and one-, two-, or three-piece inflatable cylinders (see Figure 15). The *malleable rod* implant consists of two rodlike cylinders that are implanted into the corpora cavernosa. To achieve an erection, a man manually straightens his penis into the erect position. The rods have a basic wire core that is surrounded by a polyester/silicone covering. The *semirigid rods* are made up of a series of segments held together by a central spring. A thin silicone membrane covers the entire device. The implant can easily be adjusted for length prior to insertion, but it comes in only two widths. It works in much the same way as the bendable rod implant. Sexual relations can resume 4 weeks after surgery. The *inflatable implants* provide a more natural-looking erection and are better concealed than the malleable or semirigid rod implant. There are three styles of inflatable implants: the one-, two-, or three-piece types. Since the three-piece type is the most commonly utilized inflatable penile implant, I will discuss it in detail. If you desire more information on the other two types of implants, ask your surgeon what he or she prefers to use.

The three-piece inflatable device is the Rolls-Royce of implants, combining excellent function with the most natural appearance when the penis is either flaccid or rigid. It is more complex than the other penile implants and consists of two inflatable cylinders, a pump, and a large reservoir to hold fluid. The cylinders are placed in the corpora cavernosa, the pump resides in the scrotum, and the reservoir is placed in the abdomen. The

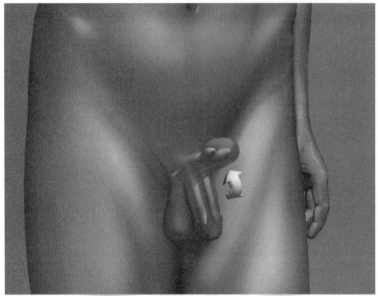

A   *malleable implant*

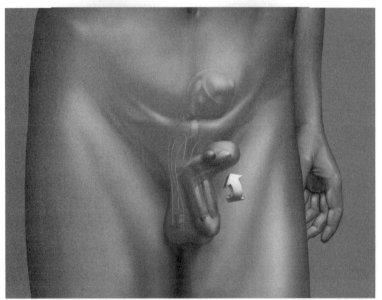

B   *inflatable implant*

Figure 15. Types of penile implants. A: A malleable implant consists of two solid cylinders. They are bent for concealment or straightened for sexual activity. B: An inflatable (in this case, three-piece) implant consists of two hollow cylinders in the penis, a pump with release valve in the scrotum, and a fluid reservoir in the abdomen.

advantage of this system over the others is that the larger reservoir holds sufficient fluid to completely fill a very large penis (see Figure 16).

This three-piece implant will last about 5 to 10 years. Anesthesia for inserting all types of implants can be local (using direct injection into and around the penis), spinal (using an injection in the lower spine to achieve anesthesia from the waist down), or general (when you go into a full sleep). You should discuss with your urologist and the hospital's anesthesiologist which is best for you. Hospital stay is usually 0 to 1 day, meaning that discharge from the hospital could take place the same day in the afternoon or the next day after an overnight stay. Recovery time is 5 to 10 days. Sexual relations can resume 4 weeks after surgery.

Postoperative Care

After surgery a urinary catheter will be left in place overnight and a cling-type dressing with mild compression is applied for 48 to 72 hours. You can take a shower after 48 to 72 hours, but you can't soak in a tub for the first 2 weeks after surgery. While you're in the hospital, you'll receive an antibiotic intravenously. After that you will continue with oral antibiotics for an additional 10 days. Immediately after surgery, the inflatable implant is left partially inflated. It is deflated either the next day, prior to discharge from the hospital, or on the first visit to your urologist. You will leave your inflatable implant deflated for about a week. Then, even though it may be uncomfortable, you will need to start inflating and deflating the implant with the help of your urologist. At the end of 4 weeks, you can resume sexual intercourse.

Chances of infection after surgery for an implant are very low (1–5%) and there is little risk of other complications. Mechanical failure of any implant continues to diminish in frequency, but there is still a problem with fluid leaking from the cylinders, requiring replacement of the part. Many implants need to be replaced after about 10 years of use.

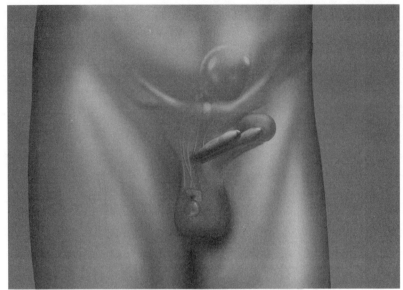

A   *inflating implant*

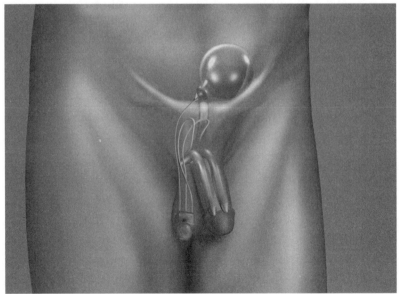

B   *deflating implant*

Figure 16. How to use a three-piece inflatable penile implant. A: The cylinders are inflated by pumping the fluid from the reservoir, creating an erection. B: The cylinders are deflated by releasing the fluid back to the reservoir, creating flaccidity.

How a three-piece inflatable implant works (Figure 16)

1. To make your penis erect, squeeze the pump (located in your scrotum) several times. This forces the fluid in the reservoir (located in your abdomen) to move from the reservoir, through the tubing, and into the cylinder in the penis. When the cylinders are full of fluid, the penis is erect.

2. To end the erection, squeeze and hold the pump's deflation valve until the fluid moves out of the cylinders and back into the reservoir. Then the penis will be in a relaxed position.

Your doctor will provide you with further detailed instructions from a brochure or video and will work with you to make sure you know how to use the implant.

TIPS FOR MAKING A TREATMENT WORK

- *Follow instructions exactly.*
- *Have a positive attitude.*
- *Practice: perfect the technique of using a mechanical device.*
- *Try an oral or injectable method or dosage at least four different times before declaring, "It doesn't work."*
- *Call your doctor if you have any questions or problems, or need encouragement.*

COST OF TREATMENT

There is an ongoing debate as to who should pay for the treatment of ED. Doctors say that it is a medical necessity, but insurance companies would like to disagree. Many insurance companies do cover the costs, but coverage varies from company to company and policy to policy. The following information is intended as a guide only and the mentioned figures are, at best, only estimates that might change from time to time and place to place.

Although insurance companies hotly debated the issue of coverage when Viagra® first became available, many companies now pay for a month's supply of Viagra® (3–6 pills). If you desire more than that, you will have to pay for each additional pill at a cost of about $10 per pill. But be sure to check around; prices vary from pharmacy to pharmacy, so you might be able to find a better price.

Vacuum pumps are generally covered by health insurance and range from $140 for the manual-pump style, $300 for a midrange style, to $500 for a deluxe electric-pump style. Alprostadil, in the injection form or suppository, costs about $18 to $32 per use. Many insurance companies cover this expense. Your health insurance company may cover all the costs of a penile implant, should you choose that treatment. Costs range from $10,000 to $15,000. Check with your insurance company prior to implant surgery. Testosterone replacement therapy is usually covered by insurance. AndroGel® costs $170 to $180 per month. Injections cost $9 to $20 per month. Sex therapy is usually not covered by insurance. Special counseling costs $50 to $300 per hour.

OTHER TREATMENTS

In some instances, surgery is required to treat damage caused by injury or trauma.

Penile revascularization (vascular surgery) is performed when there is significant damage to the major artery in the penis, causing insufficient blood to flow into the penis to create an erection. If needed, the artery is sometimes replaced in a procedure called penile arterial bypass surgery. This procedure has been available for over 20 years, yet the success rate still varies from 20 to 80 percent. This surgery is most often reserved for young patients who have had some sort of trauma or accident that has damaged this artery.

THE FUTURE: GENE THERAPY AND GROWTH FACTOR THERAPY

The most recent research for treating ED is in the field of genetics and growth factors. Scientists are hopeful that by genetically modifying a small portion of the smooth muscle cells in the penis through injection, they will be able to restore normal tissue function required for an erection. One type of gene therapy being explored has the unique advantage over other therapies in that it treats the *cause* of ED, rather than just the symptoms. Another exciting prospect of gene therapy is its lasting effects. It is potentially possible that as few as two or three penile injections per year may be all that are needed to restore the ability to attain erections. Although preclinical data in animals is encouraging for the use of gene therapy, and the future for this research seems bright, gene therapy is only in its infancy stage. Treatments will not be available even for clinical testing for several years.

QUESTIONS MY PATIENTS ASK

Q: When I drink alcohol, I feel more relaxed and sex becomes easier. Why? Does alcohol help with sex?

A: Alcohol is a drug. One of its effects is sedation. In small doses, alcohol might decrease psychological inhibitions and thus appear to increase the desire. However, it does impair the ability to generate an erection. Chronic use of alcohol, especially in large amounts, causes a condition called *neuropathy* (damage to the nerves). This in turn causes ED and, in some cases, an orgasmic disorder.

TABLE 2

Treatments at a Glance
FDA-Approved Drug Treatments for ED

BRAND NAME	CHEMICAL NAME	HOW TO TAKE
Viagra®	Sildenafil citrate	Oral tablet
Caverject®	Alprostadil sterile powder *or* Prostaglandin E_1	Injection into penis
Edex® (in United States) or Viridal® (in Europe)	Alprostadil alfadex *or* Prostaglandin E_1	Injection into penis
MUSE®	Alprostadil *or* Prostaglandin E_1	Intraurethral suppository
Uprima® or Ixense® (approved in Europe only)	Apomorphine	Tablet under the tongue

Drug Treatments for ED Being Tested

BRAND NAME	CHEMICAL NAME	HOW TO TAKE
Cialis™	Tadalafil (IC_{351})	Oral tablet
	Vardenafil	Oral tablet
Topiglan	Alprostadil *or* Prostaglandin E_1	Topical gel
Alprox-TD®	Alprostadil *or* Prostaglandin E_1	Topical gel

*Q: I read in the newspaper about this new natural treat-
ment. It doesn't need a prescription. Satisfaction guaranteed.
Should I try it?*

A: No. Although natural remedies may be appealing to you,
the great majority of them have no documented proof of being effective. If you buy this product, you will be wasting your money.
See the box "Fraud or Real?" on page 82.

*Q: I am 80 years old. Is Viagra® (or other oral medications
such as Cialis™ and Vardenafil) safe for me?*

A: If you're able to tolerate physical activities involving a
moderate level of exercise, such as climbing two flights of stairs,
and if you are not taking nitrates, it is probably safe to take
Viagra®. In elderly individuals doctors recommend that a lower
dose (for example, 25 mg) be used initially. The dosage can increase if done cautiously. Do not buy Viagra® or any other medication by yourself over the Internet or take a pill from your friend
or neighbor. Check with your doctor.

*Q: A 100 mg dose of Viagra® has not been effective for me.
Should I try 200 mg?*

A: No. Studies have shown that increasing the dose of
Viagra® from 100 mg to 200 mg does not increase its effectiveness, but does increase the side effects.

*Q: I had a heart attack 3 years ago. Is it safe to take Viagra®
or other oral medications such as Cialis™ and Vardenafil?*

A: If you're physically active, with no chest pain, if you have
been following up on your heart condition periodically with your
doctor, and if you don't take nitrates, there's no problem with
your taking Viagra®. However, before taking Viagra® or other
oral medications, check with your cardiologist to make sure that
your heart condition is stable.

Q: Medications for the treatment of ED take the spontaneity out of sex. Lovemaking has to be planned. My wife and I don't like that. What can we do?

A: Viagra®'s effectiveness for enhancing erections lasts approximately 4 hours, starting an hour after you take it. This 4-hour window leaves you enough time to be flexible and removes the pressure for immediate performance. Also, if you take Viagra® and then the sexual activity is canceled for any reason, don't be upset. No harm is done by wasting the pill. Other medications may provide other options. For example, studies have shown that the effectiveness of the new medication Cialis™ lasts up to 24 hours, thus providing longer time for spontaneity of sexual activity.

Q: What about the Viagra® death cases reported by the FDA on the Internet?

A: Unfortunately, this report has been misunderstood. The fact is that there were 130 deaths reported to the FDA in patients in whom sildenafil (Viagra®) was *prescribed*. This just means these people had a prescription for Viagra®, but *none* of these reported deaths was directly related to the use of Viagra® alone. Viagra® is an extremely well-tested and proven safe drug. For the complete report, see "Viagra and Reports of Death to the FDA," on page 143.

Q: Does having side effects of Viagra® or other oral medications such as Cialis™ and Vardenafil—headache and nasal congestion—mean that I'm at risk for other more serious complications such as heart attack?

A: No. Heart attack is not a complication of Viagra® or other oral medications. It can be triggered by any physical activity, including sexual activity. Experiencing the minor side effects of Viagra® or other oral medications does not mean you have a higher potential for serious complications.

Q: Is Viagra® currently the only effective oral medication approved by the FDA for ED?

A: Yes, but there are a number of other new medications in advanced clinical research. Approval is expected within the next few years.

Q: Can I use a vacuum device with a condom?

A: Yes, you can wear the condom after you create an erection with the vacuum device.

Q: Does surrogate therapy help?

A: There is no scientific evidence that it helps. In addition, having sex with a "surrogate" might expose you to sexually transmitted diseases. Many of the places offering surrogate therapy effectively practice masked prostitution.

Q: How many times should I try Viagra® before I give up and move on to the next treatment option?

A: Most doctors recommend at least a trial of the 100 mg dose or otherwise the highest tolerated dose on at least four different occasions. Some researchers recommend eight different occasions before declaring Viagra® ineffective.

Q: Why doesn't Viagra® work in some patients?

A: Viagra® is effective in up to 70 percent of patients with ED. The other 30 percent don't respond to Viagra® because they have severe vascular disease in the penis preventing opening of the blood vessels (vasodilation) or damage to the nerves that transmit signals to the penis.

Q: How effective are other treatments for ED after oral medications have failed?

A: Other treatments can be very effective in patients who fail with oral medications. For instance, penile self-injection therapy with medications such as Caverject® can be effective in over 80 percent of those who fail with Viagra®. Penile implants are very effective and satisfactory in those who fail with both Viagra® and injection therapy.

Q: How often can I use Viagra®?
A: A maximum of once a day.

Q: How often can I use injection therapy?
A: No more than 3 times a week and at least 24 hours between injections.

Q: How frequently can I use a penile implant?
A: As often as you want. There are no restrictions.

Q: What should I do if I get an erection lasting more than 4 hours after a penile injection?
A: Either call your doctor or go to the closest emergency room and seek an emergency consultation with a urologist. The erection will then be terminated with an antidote penile injection or other procedures. An erection lasting too long will damage the penis, because the blood that is trapped for several hours in the penis loses oxygen and nutrients and becomes toxic to the penis itself. This uncommon complication of penile injection therapy is preventable by starting at a small dose and then increasing the dose until an erection lasts for 45 to 60 minutes. Follow your doctor's dose instructions and don't increase the dose without consulting him or her.

Q: I thought once I got my erections back and I could make love to my wife again, everything would be okay in our marriage. Yet she still is cold and withdrawn from our sexual relationship. There's still a chilly distance between us. What's wrong?
A: Viagra® or other treatments will fix the "mechanical" problem of sex, but it does not fix the psychological or relation-

ship problems. You should ask your doctor to refer you to a marriage counselor or sex therapist and resolve your relationship problems. It will be worth the effort.

Q: I'm considering surgery to have an inflatable implant. How can I be sure that just bumping into things or lying on my stomach at the beach won't suddenly make the implant inflate?

A: Don't worry. Your implant is securely in place in your body and can't inflate itself. In order to inflate it, you have to compress the pump from two sides. Pressure on just one side of the pump won't inflate the implant, so lying on your stomach or bumping into something won't do anything.

Q: I'm uncomfortable about trying injection therapy. Is sticking a needle into my penis painful?

A: The idea of injection therapy sounds very strange and scary to most of my patients. A man naturally fears inserting a needle into his penis. However, when my patients receive their first injection, they are usually pleasantly surprised. The needle stick itself is either painless or minimally painful. As a point of reference, most people know the pain of needles from drawing blood during blood tests. The majority of my patients report that penile self-injection therapy is significantly less painful than the needles of blood tests.

Q: Will anyone be able to see my penile implant and know that I have one?

A: No. An implant is completely inside your body. If you walked around naked, nobody would be able to see your implant.

Q: How long does an erection of an inflatable penile implant last?

A: As long as you want. You decide when to inflate the implant (i.e., start an erection) and you decide when to deflate the implant (i.e., terminate the erection).

Q: If, for any reason, I don't like my penile implant, can I have it removed?

A: Technically, yes. But removing the penile implant usually causes scar tissue to develop in the penis and the penis may shrink. A patient planning to have a penile implant should be committed to this treatment option for life. You should go into surgery realizing that this is a permanent treatment, similar to other implants in the body—like a hip joint, knee joint, or pacemaker.

Q: If I develop an infection and my penile implant has to be removed, what are my options?

A: You could have another implant in 3 to 6 months after the removal of the infected one. Sometimes, I perform a "salvage procedure" in which I remove the original implant and immediately reimplant a new one. However, if no other implant is inserted, you can use a vacuum device. Other treatment options such as oral medications or injection therapy will no longer be successful.

Q: When could I go back to work after a penile implant surgery?
A: In 5 to 10 days.

Q: When can I have sex after a penile implant?
A: In 4 to 6 weeks.

Q: Viagra® alone is not adequate. Can I combine Viagra® and Caverject®?

A: No. Don't do that on your own. Consult your doctor, and if he recommends combination therapy, then do it under supervision. Thus far, very few studies have addressed the issues of effectiveness and safety of combination therapies. However, in the next few years I expect we'll see more research of various different combinations.

Q: I'm 60 years old and have had ED for 3 years. Since the most common cause of ED is vascular disease, is penile vascular surgery appropriate for me?

A: Penile revascularization is an appropriate treatment option only for a very small number of patients with ED. The best candidates are usually young, otherwise-healthy men who have ED following a pelvic fracture or trauma causing injury to the penile arteries. Although the most common cause of ED is vascular, penile revascularization is not indicated because the vascular disease causing ED frequently causes dysfunction of the end organ, i.e., the penis.

Q: What are the restrictions after a penile implant?

A: There really are no restrictions. Even biking and horseback riding are permitted after a penile implant, with some precautions. When biking, a man with a penile implant should wear padded sports shorts and avoid narrow, hard bike seats—use wide, padded seats instead. These shorts are also recommended for horseback riding. Just avoid bumping trauma on the perineum.

Q: Since I had treatment for my ED, I have been unsure about how satisfied I am. Part of having sex is the enjoyment of "me being able." Although I am now "able," frequently I feel that it is the pill or the injection that is "able" and not me. Honestly, my partner frequently feels the same way. She tells me, "it is the treatment, it is not you!"

A: I would like to assure you that it is still *you* and not the pill, the injection, or even your penile implant. *You* are the one who initiates the treatment, *you* are the one who desires it, and *you* are the one who controls it. I have discussed this important issue with many of my patients and their partners. Many patients and partners have found ways to handle this. You may want to think about your ED treatment the same way you think about your eyeglasses. It is not your eyeglasses that see, it is *you* who see and read. If you or your partner feels strongly about this issue, bring it up with your doctor. He or she might be able to help you by choosing the treatment option that best addresses this issue. Remember that different treatment options offer different features, such as onset of action, duration of action, route of administration, etc. Work with your doctor to choose the treatment that not only works mechanically, but also addresses all your and your partner's needs and feelings. In addition, you might want to consult with a sex therapist to help with this or similar issues.

VI

Prostate Cancer and ED

———————————— ▬ ————————————

The harshest onset of ED comes with facing the reality of prostate cancer. One day you are healthy (or so you think), and the next day, after a standard yearly physical and a blood test for the prostate-specific antigen (PSA), you find out you have cancer. Your first reaction and that of your sexual partner will be to "get through it, save your life, fight the cancer, and get rid of it—nothing else matters." But something else does matter, especially to you: your sexual well-being, your ability to have an erection. Although you cannot ignore the prostate cancer, any of the various treatments for it can rob you of your sexual ability. And once the cancer threat is passed, and you know you'll survive and you get your normal life back, sexual performance will suddenly be very important again. Facing ED as a result of prostate cancer treatment can be devastating, but let me reassure you that there *is* treatment that will work for you if normal function does not spontaneously return.

Prostate cancer is increasing as the population of the United States grows older. In 2000 it was estimated that about 180,400 cases of prostate cancer were diagnosed in the United States, and 31,900 men died of this disease. Fortunately, this cancer progresses slowly, and is easily detected, so it can be diagnosed and treated early on. A routine part of a yearly physical now involves a digital rectal exam and a blood test to check the serum levels of prostate-specific antigen (PSA). When prostate cancer is detected early, it can be treated and totally removed from your body, curing you of the disease.

TREATMENTS FOR LOCALIZED PROSTATE CANCER

If and when you are diagnosed with prostate cancer, there are a variety of treatments available. Unfortunately, all of the treatments can affect your sexual function sooner or later. But remember, you must first rid your body of the cancer, then you and your doctor can address sexual difficulties. If your cancer is localized (confined only to the prostate), there are three standard treatments available for your consideration.

Watchful Waiting

This treatment is a passive treatment and may be the best option for older men who have a complicated medical history and already have several other illnesses that may cause their death before the prostate cancer even becomes a major threat. It is also an option for older men who have a very small tumor and choose to watch carefully to determine whether it increases in size or remains the same. Since prostate cancer is often a slow-progressing cancer, this passive treatment may be possible.

Radiation Therapy

External radiation treatment burns out the cancer in the prostate gland. As it burns out the cancerous cells, it causes scar tissue (fibrosis) to form. This scar tissue destroys the arteries (vascular structure) and the nerves surrounding the prostate that are crucial for relaying blood flow and "messages" to the penis to create an erection. As these critical arteries and nerves are gradually destroyed by the radiation, your erections will weaken and eventually (over about 1 to 3 years) you might have complete ED. The volume of your ejaculation will also be less and more watery since the prostate creates the "juice" for ejaculation.

The advantages of radiation treatment are:

1. It doesn't require surgery or blood loss.
2. It can be done on an outpatient basis. Visits to the hospital are brief.
3. Sexual function will continue during treatment.
4. Ejaculation is possible although weak and watery after treatment.

The disadvantages include:

1. Uncertainty about killing off all the cancer cells.
2. The possibility of development of new prostate cancer, because the prostate gland is not removed.
3. Diarrhea and urinary frequency as side effects of radiation.
4. Erectile function diminished or lost after 1 to 2 years of treatment.

Brachytherapy is an internal form of radiation therapy in which radioactive "seeds" are implanted into the prostate to destroy the cancer cells. Effects are similar to external radiation therapy.

Surgery

This treatment is the one most commonly recommended to men who have localized prostate cancer and a reasonable life expectancy. Radical prostatectomy is the procedure in which the prostate and a small rim of tissue around the gland are completely removed with the intent to ensure that 100 percent of all cancerous cells have been removed. This surgery may sound aggressive, but it has the advantage of curing you of the cancer while preserving the quality of your life.

Your surgeon will make every attempt to spare the nerves that surround the prostate in order to ensure your recovery of sexual function (see Figure 17). In some cases the nerves can remain intact and be pushed aside during the removal of the prostate. This procedure is called *bilateral nerve-sparing technique* since the nerves on both sides of the prostate are spared. Men who undergo this procedure have a 40 to 80 percent (average 60 percent) chance of regaining complete erectile function in 12 to 24 months as the nerves slowly recover from the shock of surgery.

If the cancer, however, is bulging to one side, the surgeon must cut the nerve on that side of the gland to remove it. This procedure is called *unilateral nerve-sparing technique* since the nerves on one side of the prostate are spared. Men who undergo this procedure have a 20 to 40 percent (average 30 percent) chance of regaining complete erectile function in 12 to 24 months.

If the cancer is bulging on both sides of the gland, the surgeon must cut the nerves on both sides of the prostate. There are instances where all the nerves surrounding the prostate must be cut to remove the gland. This is called *bilateral nerve resection.* In this instance, the patient will rarely regain erectile function.

For those patients who require loss of the penile nerves on one or both sides, there is a new surgical technique under development. It involves a nerve graft. During radical prostatectomy, a piece of a nerve in the leg, called the sural nerve, is harvested and transplanted to the pelvis after removal of the prostate. This nerve graft will function as a conduit for regeneration of the penile nerves. This procedure is currently under development in a number of major university centers, including our Department of Urology at Columbia University. Early results are encouraging.

A major review of the medical literature reveals that the rate of normal erectile function, after all types of radical prostatectomy by a variety of surgeons, was 42 percent. After nerve-sparing radical prostatectomy, whether or not you regain erectile function is also determined by your age: the younger you are, the better your chance of regaining complete function. On the other hand, if you experienced partial ED before surgery, you have a lower chance of regaining sexual function after surgery.

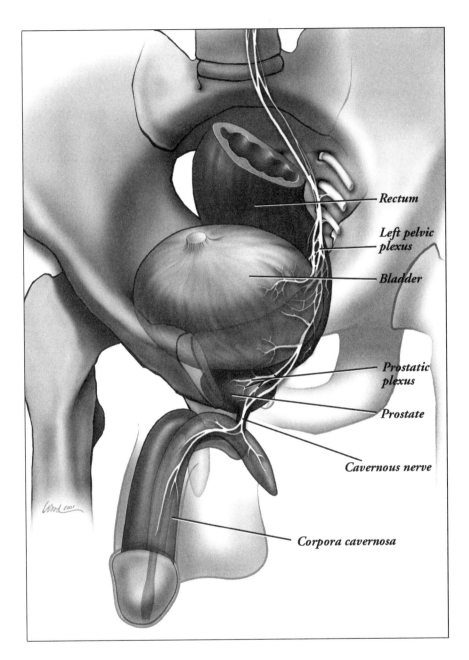

Figure 17. The anatomy of the penile nerves in relationship to the prostate. The nerves responsible for erection originate in the spinal cord in the lower back and extend to the penis, passing just on the right and left sides of the prostate.

Before surgery your surgeon will not be able to guarantee that he or she will be able to use a nerve-sparing technique. The primary goal of prostate surgery is to remove all of the cancer. If the cancer is localized in the prostate and is successfully removed, you will no longer have any threat of cancer from the prostate gland. Your surgeon is first concerned with saving your life and making you cancer-free. His or her second priority is to spare any nerves possible to ensure you every chance of normal sexual function.

Advantages of surgery:

- Cancer is completely removed.
- Spontaneous erectile function may resume after 12 to 24 months.
- Treatment is quick; it is over and done with.
- Orgasm is still possible.

Disadvantages of surgery:

- There is blood loss and a small chance of incontinence.
- The hospital stay is 2 to 4 days, and recovery takes 4 to 8 weeks.
- Ejaculation is no longer possible.

Cryotherapy. This therapy is the last option for treating localized prostate cancer. It's currently used for localized advanced prostate cancer if and when radiation therapy fails. This procedure uses liquid nitrogen to freeze the prostate, killing the prostate, the cancer cells and the nerves surrounding the gland. Although this process can be lifesaving, ED is an inevitable result almost 100 percent of the time.

TREATMENT FOR ADVANCED PROSTATE CANCER

Hormone Therapy

This therapy is used in cases of advanced prostate cancer in which the cancer has spread to the bones and/or other organs. Hormone therapy does not cure the cancer, but it does slow down its progress and ease the pain associated with it. These medications reduce the levels of testosterone in the blood by stopping the testicles from producing testosterone. Since prostate cancer grows under the influence of the male hormones, stopping the production of this hormone in the body reduces the prostate cancer or slows it down. This palliative therapy is used only in cases of advanced cancer that has spread to other parts of the body. Most patients with advanced cancer are older. This therapy causes a majority of patients to have erectile dysfunction, low sex drive, and an inability to reach orgasm.

RESUMING SEX AFTER PROSTATE SURGERY

As with most major operations, prostate surgery will require you to be in the hospital from 2 to 4 days. A full recovery sometimes takes up to 4 weeks and maybe up to 8 weeks. While you were facing the death threat of having cancer, you, like most of my patients, were probably not too concerned about your sex life. Your primary concern was your entire life and how many more years you would have to live. Now that you've successfully overcome the threat of cancer and are starting to feel better after the surgery, your thoughts start turning to the question, "Will I ever be able to make love again?" I can answer that question with an emphatic, "Yes, of course you will." If you encounter ED in the early months after surgery, there is still a possibility that normal function will resume in about 12 to 24 months. And even if you face ED during or beyond that amount of time, there are many treatments available to you (see Chapter V). With the use of these treatments, the large majority of men with ED after radical prostatectomy can resume a satisfactory sex life.

As you start feeling better after surgery, begin being intimate again with your partner (see Chapter IX) to reestablish the physical and emotional closeness you had prior to surgery. Celebrate together the fact that you've been victorious over cancer! Anticipate that you will soon regain the ability to have an erection. Ask your doctor if you can use Viagra® or injection therapy while you are waiting for normal function to return. According to *The Journal of Urology*, the use of penile self-injection therapy is very helpful in keeping the penis "alive and active" while the nerves in the area of the removed prostate regenerate themselves and spontaneous erections return. Studies have shown that Viagra® was most effective in patients who had bilateral nerve-sparing technique (72%), less effective in those who had unilateral nerve-sparing (50%), and least effective, or ineffective, in those who had bilateral nerve resection (15%). However, even if Viagra® is not effective right after surgery, it may be successful later on, so keep trying periodically—probably every 3 months.

With the introduction of Viagra® and its effective results, people started talking about ED and admitting they had the problem. Former senator and presidential candidate Bob Dole, who developed erectile problems as a side effect of prostate surgery, was one of the first well-known individuals to speak openly about their ED and treatment. Dole kept his suffering private until he successfully used Viagra®. He was so pleased and excited by the results that he became an advocate for the medication and a spokesman for ED. He began urging men with similar problems to pay attention to their health and investigate their options.

If Viagra® or other oral medications are not effective, don't put off having sex. It is important to continue to be sexually active, or in other words to "exercise" the penis after the prostate surgery. This is thought to give you the best chance of return function. Some researchers believe that erections enhance tissue oxygenation and suppress smooth muscle fibrosis (scarring). Until the nerves regenerate or recover sufficiently to respond to Viagra®, injection therapy is the most effective and reliable way of restoring erectile function. A recent study showed that injection therapy can aid erections soon after surgery to increase the chances of the return of normal function. In patients who had nerve-sparing radical prostatectomy, initiation of injection therapy soon after the prostate surgery improved the return of spontaneous erections from a dismal 20 percent to a promising 50 to 70 percent!

In some cases no erectile function will return after even 24 months. In that case, spontaneous sexual function will probably never come back. At this point you may want to explore the option of a penile implant as a permanent solution to your ED.

After prostate surgery, you will be able to achieve orgasm; however, you will have no ejaculation, since the prostate is no longer available to produce the fluid.

Viagra® has also been shown to be effective in patients who had external radiation therapy and brachytherapy to treat their prostate cancer.

A diagnosis of prostate cancer is not a death sentence for you or your love life. Effective treatment and/or surgery will eliminate the cancer if it is contained in the prostate and extend your lifetime. A wide variety of treatment options will guarantee you a love life, even if you do not regain spontaneous function.

QUESTIONS MY PATIENTS ASK

Q. Now that the threat of cancer is passed, I feel like I've sold off my right to sex for the right to live, and that makes me angry. How can I resolve these feelings?

A: By obtaining the proper treatment for ED, the majority of men can have satisfactory erections and a quality sex life after the treatment of prostate cancer. Learn more about the effects of the prostate cancer treatments on your sexual function. Read up on the treatments for erectile dysfunction in general. There is hope. There are solutions. Don't simply give up.

Q: Can my doctor tell me ahead of time what type of nerve-sparing surgery will have to take place?

A: Probably not. Your surgeon will not know for sure the position and extent of the cancer until performing surgery. He or she will spare the nerves if at all possible, but the primary goal is to rid you of every cancer cell.

Q: How can you say I'll regain normal sex function after removal of the prostate when I won't be able to ejaculate anymore? To me that's part of being "normal."

A: You'll be able to have satisfactory erections either spontaneously or aided by a treatment for ED—that's normal. You'll be able to reach orgasm, which is the climax of pleasurable excitement—that's normal. But your orgasm won't be associated with ejaculations, which is the ejection of fluid semen. Many patients (and doctors) nickname this "dry orgasms." In spite of that, the majority of patients and partners are able to enjoy their sex life with the proper education and treatment.

Q: My wife is so afraid that I won't be able to "perform" and that it will embarrass me, she doesn't even want to attempt sex. What should we do?

A: I can assure you and your wife that after your treatment

for prostate cancer, you will be able to maintain or regain your erections; or you will be able to find a treatment that will assure you of erections. All of the options will lead you and your wife to an enjoyable sex life with satisfactory erections. Stay close to each other and follow up with your doctor about your concerns.

Q: *How will I know that my normal sexual function has returned?*

A: Don't worry—it won't hide itself. You'll start seeing your morning erections and erections from sexual stimulation gradually improve.

Q: *Is there any way the surgeon can reconnect the nerves around the prostate after removing the gland so that I can have a normal erection right away?*

A: This is a great idea that is presently being pursued by some surgeons. Their pioneering work includes "harvesting" a nerve from the lower leg and grafting it to the cut nerves near the prostate at the time of a radical prostatectomy. This surgery is currently under development in several centers in the United States, including our Department of Urology at Columbia University in New York City. In a team approach, I participate with the urologist performing the removal of the prostate, to perform the nerve graft procedure when needed.

Q: *Why does it take so long (up to 24 months) to know whether or not I'll have normal erections again?*

A: Nerves grow back (regenerate) at a rate of ½ inch per month—a very slow process. Only after the nerves have grown and reconnected will you be able to have spontaneous erections again.

Q: *I had radical prostatectomy three months ago. I've regained my bladder control but still don't have erections. Why?*

A: "Connectors" or nerves that are disturbed during

prostate surgery that supply the bladder and the sphincter muscle are different from those that supply the penis. The bladder "connectors" or nerves and the sphincter muscle probably heal faster than the others. But don't worry. Your normal erections will probably return within a year or so.

Q: My brother had radical prostatectomy for prostate cancer three years ago and he uses injection therapy for ED. Since I also had radical prostatectomy and have ED, should I try some of his injections?

A: No, never try the penile injection of someone else, because the dose is very individualized. Your brother's dose might be an overdose for you or vice versa. In order to avoid priapism (prolonged erection), doctors start injection therapy at a small dose for all patients and then increase the dose until a satisfactory response is reached, requiring different doses for different patients. Talk to your doctor or a urologist to find out your options and if injection therapy is right for you.

VII

Heart Disease and ED

SEXUAL ACTIVITY AND HEART FUNCTION

The physical exertion on the heart caused by sexual activity has often been compared to other normal physical activities such as walking or running, or to the emotional states of anger or fear. The effects of orgasm on the heart, blood pressure, and oxygen consumed are only a little greater than the effects during sexual arousal. There can be some differences owing to individual circumstances surrounding the sexual activity: type of sexual stimulation, familiarity with partner, intercourse position, and food and/or alcohol consumption. But in general, sexual activity is similar to mild or moderate exercise for most individuals with or without coronary artery disease. Heart rate during sex rarely increases to 130 beats per minute and the systolic (upper value) blood pressure rarely exceeds 170. In fact, your normal daily physical activities are more strenuous on your heart than any sexual activity, including intercourse and orgasm.

> *The risk of heart attack during or after sex is only slightly higher than playing a round of golf.*

A standard way of measuring physical exertion is MET (metabolic equivalent of energy expenditure at the resting state). MET values have been assigned to a variety of daily activities. For example, walking at 2 miles per hour is assigned an energy expenditure of 2 METs. Sexual activity is given 2 to 3 METs prior to orgasm, and 3 to 4 METs during orgasm. Some younger people have reached 5 to 6 METs during sex, but the lower range is the norm for older individuals or those in long-established relationships.

Fewer than 1% of heart attacks occur during sex. A 50-year-old man in the United States has a baseline yearly risk of heart attack of about 1%. This risk increases only slightly to 1.01% during sexual activity. Even a high-risk man who has had a previous heart attack has only a 1.10% risk of a heart attack during sex.

TREATMENT OF ED IN PATIENTS WITH HEART DISEASE

The chance of ED occurring in men with cardiovascular disease is significantly higher than that in the general population. ED occurring in a male who was previously fine may indicate that he has a possible risk of coronary artery disease. This is not to say that every man who has ED should run out and have an EKG test. Rather it should be taken as a precaution. If you have other cardiac symptoms and/or risk factors as well as ED, you should point this out to your doctor since ED and cardiovascular disease share many of the same risk factors and frequently occur together.

Patients believed to be at risk for heart disease are classified into low-, indeterminate-, and high-risk categories. The large majority of patients are in the *low-risk* category. This includes those with:

- Controlled high blood pressure
- Mild, stable (being treated) angina (chest pain), not taking any nitrate-containing medications

---

RISK FACTORS FOR HEART DISEASE

- *Age*
- *Male; postmenopausal female*
- *High blood pressure*
- *Diabetes*
- *Obesity*
- *Cigarette smoking*
- *High cholesterol*
- *Family history of heart disease*
- *Sedentary lifestyle*

Patients with three or more risk factors (other than gender) are considered to be at a slightly increased risk during sex.

Source: Advice from the Princeton Consensus Conference, July 2000.

- Successful heart bypass surgery (revascularization)
- A history of uncomplicated heart attack (myocardial infarction, MI), more than 6 weeks previous
- Mild disease of heart valves
- No symptoms of heart disease and fewer than three cardiovascular risk factors
- Class I congestive heart failure (see New York Heart Association classifications in the below box)

The New York Heart Association has four different classifications of congestive heart failure:

Class I: those with heart disease who experience ordinary physical activity without breathlessness.

Class II: those with heart disease who experience shortness of breath during some activity such as brisk walking.

Class III: those with heart disease who experience breathlessness with even slight activity such as walking on a flat surface.

Class IV: those with heart disease who are breathless even while resting.

If you are in the low-risk category, you can initiate and resume sexual activity and seek treatment for ED if needed under the supervision of your doctor. It is important to continue with routine checkups, every 6 to 12 months and to monitor your risks for heart disease.

Note: If you are taking a nitrate medication for your heart condition, you cannot take Viagra® or other PDE-5 inhibitors. Taking Viagra® or other PDE-5 inhibitors with a nitrate can cause your blood pressure to plunge to a life-threatening low level. Choose an alternate treatment for your ED.

Nitrates are found in many prescription drugs that treat chest pain caused by heart disease, such as:

• Nitroglycerin in various forms: sprays, ointments, skin patches, pastes, and tablets

• Isosorbide mononitrate and isosorbide dinitrate: tablets that are chewed, swallowed, or allowed to dissolve in your mouth

• Recreational drugs such as amyl nitrate or nitrite ("poppers")

Those individuals in the *indeterminate-risk* category include those with:

- Moderate, stable angina
- A recent heart attack (less than 6 weeks prior)
- Left ventricle dysfunction and/or Class II congestive heart failure
- Nonsustained low-risk irregular heartbeat (arrhythmia)
- Three or more risk factors for coronary artery disease (other than gender)

If you are in this category, you should undergo additional evaluation and specialized cardiac testing such as treadmill exercise stress test, to determine if you will be classified in the high-risk category or return to the low-risk category.

Men in the *high-risk* category include those with:

- Angina that is unstable or resistant to treatment
- Uncontrolled hypertension
- Class III or IV congestive heart failure or left ventricle dysfunction
- Very recent heart attack (less than 2 weeks) or stroke
- High-risk irregular heartbeat (arrhythmia)
- A disease or weakness in the heart muscle (cardiomyopathy)
- Moderate to severe heart valve disease

If you are in this high-risk group, your doctor will want to stabilize your cardiac condition with specialized treatment. Your heart condition needs to be completely evaluated, treated, and stabilized before you can resume any sexual activity or get treated for ED.

> *Important Notice: If you are using Viagra® or other PDE-5 inhibitors for ED and suddenly experience chest pains or other signs of a heart attack, seek medical attention immediately. However, be sure to tell the paramedics or attending physician at the emergency room what you are taking and the time of your last medication. This is important to avoid receiving treatment with nitrates, because the combination of Viagra® and other PDE-5 inhibitors and nitrate is dangerous.*

RESUMING SEX AFTER A HEART ATTACK

Although it is common for men who have had a heart attack (myocardial infarction or MI) or coronary artery bypass surgery to experience ED, they and their partners should not succumb to the notion that they can never resume their normal sex life. Decrease in sexual desire and ED caused by various heart medications can be addressed. Usually, the couple has a greater concern: the fear that the exertion from engaging in sexual intercourse will cause another heart attack. Sadly, because of this fear, over 50 percent of all post–heart attack and post–coronary artery bypass patients never resume a satisfactory sexual life. That need not happen. The fear of inducing another heart attack while having sex may be real, but in a fit patient with good tolerance of physical exercise, the risk is low. In fact, various research studies show that having sex or reaching an orgasm is no more strenuous than any other moderate exercise. There is no reason for you not to be able to resume sexual activity 6 to 8 weeks after having a heart attack. Some patients, who have successfully completed a stress test, may be allowed to resume sex after only 3 to 4 weeks. Check with your heart doctor with any concerns about sexual activity and your heart.

> There is a high incidence of ED with the use of Digoxin. This heart medication causes the blood vessels to contract, and contraction is the opposite of what is needed to attain an erection. An erection requires relaxation of tissues and dilation of the blood vessels. However, if you are taking Digoxin and experiencing ED, do not stop Digoxin on your own. Check first with your cardiologist, and also ask about your options for the treatment of ED.

Here are the facts from one study completed in 1996, reported in the *Journal of the American Medical Association*:

- The risk of heart attack in a healthy 50-year-old man in the United States is 1 percent per year, or 1 per million men per hour.
- The relative risk of a heart attack occurring during sex or within 2 hours after sex is 2.5 times higher than the risk of a heart attack when not having sex.
- In men who have had a heart attack, the risk of a repeat heart attack during or after sex is 2.9 times higher than the risk of

a heart attack when not having sex (not much more significant than the risk of heart attack in healthy men during or after sex).

There are, however, other risk factors that can trigger another heart attack. Extreme anger doubles your risk, and extreme physical activity (like shoveling snow) in someone with a sedentary lifestyle increases the risk of another heart attack! Your risk of having a heart attack during or after sex, whether or not you've already had heart problems, is low. And besides that, a study suggested that sex with your spouse is less risky than extramarital sex. I encourage you to not use your heart condition as an excuse for putting off your sexual activity. Talk to your doctor!

Now, if I still haven't convinced you, here's something else you can do to test out your endurance for yourself. Ask your doctor to order a treadmill exercise stress test for you and be sure your partner can watch. If you can tolerate a moderate amount of effort on the treadmill, you can tolerate sex. The effort on the treadmill is the equivalent of what your heart will experience during sex (4 to 5 METs). The treadmill exam should help relieve some of your fear and your partner's anxiety.

Another thing you can do to regain confidence about handling the exertion of sex is to exercise regularly by walking daily and "working up a sweat" at least three times a week. It's a proven fact that regular exercise is (in medical terms) a risk modifier. The chance of having a heart attack during or after sexual activity is reduced if you exercise regularly. So here's a great incentive to get out there and walk—it will improve your sex life! Of course, if you have heart problems, be sure to check with your doctor before beginning any form of exercise, just to be safe. Don't overdo it on that first outing. Take it slow at first, then gradually walk a little farther and/or a little faster. You should always be able to carry on a conversation while you're walking without feeling breathless. So get out there and walk. Start today. Your general health and mental attitude will improve while you prove to yourself (and your partner) that you are ready to resume your sex life.

> *Only 1 percent of all heart attacks occur during or shortly after having sex.*

Don't let your unfounded fears of a heart attack stop you from enjoying life to the fullest. If you've had heart problems and are now suffering from ED, talk to your doctor, address the problem, and start treatment. Don't let your heart *disease* stop you from following your heart's *desire*.

QUESTIONS MY PATIENTS ASK

Q: The wife asks: My husband has angina (chest pain). Can he take Viagra®?

A: Angina frequently is a symptom of heart disease or more accurately a symptom of coronary artery disease that requires an evaluation by a cardiologist. Angina is commonly treated with nitrate medications (coronary vasodilators) that cannot be taken with Viagra® or other medications of the PDE-5 inhibitors class. The combination of nitrate medication and Viagra® causes a dangerous drop in blood pressure and can result in death. If your husband has angina, he should first see a cardiologist for evaluation and treatment of his heart disease before trying to treat his ED. Once his heart disease is stabilized and he is permitted to resume sex, then he can look into the treatment options for his ED. If he's not taking nitrate medications, he can be a candidate for Viagra® or other PDE-5 inhibitors. But if he's taking nitrates, he'll have to consider other treatments.

VIAGRA® AND REPORTS OF DEATH TO THE FDA

The Food and Drug Administration (FDA) maintains a website for all reports of death in association with any drug. This does not necessarily mean that the drug caused the death; it just means that a person was on that drug when he died. In other words, if you are taking a cold medication and die, someone could report that fact on the FDA website, even though there was no connection between the medication and your cause of death.

Here are the facts:

Between March 1998 and mid-November 1998, 6 million men were given prescriptions for Viagra® in the United States. Of those 6 million:

• 130 deaths were reported to the FDA of patients who had a prescription for Viagra®.

• 2 deaths were due to homicide and drowning.

• 16 to 19 men who died may have taken a nitrate in combination with Viagra®.

• 44 of the 128 (34%) had onset of symptoms, or death, within 4 to 5 hours after taking Viagra®.

• 90 of the 128 (70%) had one or more risk factors for heart disease, high blood pressure, high cholesterol, diabetes, smoked cigarettes, were overweight, or had a history of heart disease. The cause of death in these men has not been clearly identified, but there is no evidence that Viagra® was the cause.

• No deaths were directly related to the use of Viagra® alone.

To give these statistics some perspective, if we were to use the Centers for Disease Control study data, the expected death rate for a general population of 6 million people (not receiving Viagra®) would be more than 2,500 individuals per week!

For the FDA's clinical information on Viagra® see:
www.fda.gov/cder/news/ viagra.htm.

Q: *I have sublingual (under-the-tongue) nitroglycerin on a standby or as-needed basis. It's been two years since I last needed to take one. I've read that the combination of Viagra® and nitroglycerin is really bad. Is it okay to take Viagra®? I promise I'll never take Viagra® and nitroglycerin together!*

A: I recommend that anyone who has nitrate medications in any form or dose not take Viagra® or any other PDE-5 inhibitors. This applies to your situation. Check with your cardiologist to see if you still need to carry nitroglycerin on a standby basis. If he or she decides you need nitroglycerin just in case, you shouldn't have Viagra®. If you don't need nitroglycerin, then discontinue carrying it and try Viagra® or any other PDE-5 inhibitors.

Q: *Is Viagra® safe in a patient with a pacemaker?*

A: Generally yes, when the patient has a stable condition and is able to tolerate physical activities. But it's a good rule to consult with your cardiologist if you have any doubt.

VIII

For Women Only:
Your Role in ED

───────•━━━•───────

ED is not just a man's problem or a woman's problem. ED is a couple's problem. Although the male may have some physical condition that needs to be addressed, it is always best if the couple is involved in every step of the acknowledgment, diagnosis, and treatment of ED. There is a far greater success rate in treatment if both partners are actively involved in understanding all aspects of ED. A couple's participation also enhances communication, establishes a more accurate sexual history, and reduces stress and anxiety for everyone involved.

YOUR ROLE IN UNDERSTANDING

If and when your partner experiences erectile dysfunction, he feels that he has failed, that his masculinity is being threatened, that he is no longer in control. These feelings are very frightening to a man. As his lack of performance continues, he may be ashamed, or anxious, or insecure, not only in the bedroom but also in other aspects of his life. As his insecurity grows, he may become depressed. Depression is quite common in men with ED, leading to a further decline in their quality of life.

You and your partner should understand, however, that

aging does bring on some changes in sexual performance. These changes are normal and should not be considered a sign of inadequacy.

Normal aging signs related to male sexual function are:

- It takes longer to achieve an erection.
- Stronger stimulation is needed to achieve an erection.
- Erection is weaker and of shorter duration.
- The time it takes to achieve a second erection is longer.
- Spontaneous erections occur less frequently.

With patience, understanding, and communication, you and your partner can continue to enjoy sex for many years. Should your partner be faced with ED, you need to work on that situation together. Too many couples do not take the time to calmly and quietly talk about this joint problem.

> As men age, they need stronger physical stimulation to achieve an erection.

I'm always somewhat surprised when I ask my patients, "Have you talked to your wife about this?" and their reply is, "No." Since I know men have a hard time expressing their feelings, even to their wives, let me share with you some of the replies I get to a series of routine questions I ask.

Q: *How often do you think about your sexual problem?*
A: Oh, almost constantly. Knowing I can't perform makes me feel like I've lost my power. I just can't get used to the idea. I feel like a part of me has died. I don't feel complete.

Q: *Has your problem affected your self-image?*
A: I used to feel in control of myself; now I feel I've lost control . . . not just of this, but of everything. I feel like I've lost my manhood.

Q: Are you sexually attracted to your wife?

A: Oh, yes. I find her very attractive, but I avoid approaching her sexually since I know I'm going to fail. I won't be able to perform and that's just too painful for me to face. So, I avoid it altogether.

Q: How has your partner reacted to your ED?

A: I think she's very understanding. She just doesn't bring up the subject. I think she just doesn't want to hurt my feelings, or maybe, I really don't know, but maybe she doesn't have any sexual interest in me anymore.

Q: Do you think your wife is interested in sex?

A: I don't know. We rarely talk about it. Probably she's not interested. I guess to really know I would have to ask her directly.

Q: How has your ED affected the quality of your life?

A: It has made me depressed. Every time I can't get it up, I realize I'm getting older, that my body is failing me—first this, then something else. What's next to fail—my heart? And pow, it's all over.

I'm anxious about trying anything for fear I'll fail. I used to be good at sex; now I fail at it regularly. It makes me wonder what else I'll suddenly start failing at.

Q: Have you talked to anyone about your ED?

A: No. Nobody at all. Are you kidding? I could hardly get up the nerve to tell you about it. No way would I ever admit this to a friend.

Your partner's sexual function is very important to him. Sex is extremely important to most men throughout their lives, no matter what their age. Although your interest in sex may wane, his does not. To ignore or deemphasize the importance of sex in your relationship can cause your partner to feel alienated from you and your relationship. Be sure to communicate with your partner how you feel about sex. Explain to him what your sexual desires and needs are. He may be in the dark about how you feel. Don't let a lack of communication, as well as ED, push you farther apart.

In addition, you will need to do the following:

Understand the problem: Read up on and familiarize yourself with information on ED.

Understand the anatomy and physiology behind an erection: how it works, and what hinders it from working.

Understand the diagnosis: Since there are many aspects of ED, be sure you completely understand the diagnosis that the doctor gives. If at all possible, go to the doctor with your partner so together you can understand what is going on.

Understand your options: There may be several options for how your partner's ED can be treated. Be sure you understand what the treatments are and how they work.

Understand the treatment: When your doctor prescribes a treatment, make sure you and your spouse clearly understand how to use the treatment, the side effects of the treatment, the advantages and disadvantages of the treatment, and what to expect for results from the treatment.

YOUR ROLE IN COMMUNICATION

It is of utmost importance that you talk about sexual problems with your partner. To ignore a problem and live in silence will only worsen the situation. However, the first time your partner can't attain or maintain an erection is not the time to rush in and seek medical attention. Remember, the definition of ED specifies that the condition must persist over a period of time. "So how should I respond?" you might ask. Here are a few things you can say that will reassure your partner and convey your understanding:

"I love you."

"We can find a way to handle this problem. This is a medical
    condition and it's treatable."

"Sex is our joint project. We enjoy it together, and if there are
    problems with it, we can solve them together."

"I care about you and how you are feeling."

"I read that difficulty having an erection can have a number
    of causes—physical, psychological, or a combination of
    the two. Don't worry, I'll work with you. We'll get this
    problem solved and get the best treatment for it."

Don't be critical or place blame. Don't say or imply that it
doesn't matter, because it really does matter to him. Remember
there might be an obvious cause for this nonperformance that can
easily be rectified if you ask for help.

DO'S AND DON'TS IN COMMUNICATION

Do:

Be understanding.

Give it time (at least 3 months).

Love often.

Be supportive and loving.

Say, "We can work this out together."

Offer to go with him to the doctor.

Read up on the subject of ED.

Share any knowledge about ED with your partner.

Don't:

Criticize.

Take the blame (it's not your fault).

Think he doesn't love you.

Stop being affectionate.

Avoid the issue (silence will make it worse).

Accept excuses.

If and when you seek help together, communication with your partner's doctor will be very important. Agree ahead of time which one of you will be providing the critical information to the doctor. If your partner is uncomfortable talking about ED, by all means you should be the spokesperson for the facts; however, your partner needs to share his feelings and desires on his own. Clearly communicate to your doctor what you as a couple are expecting from treatment. If your doctor orders some tests, make sure you follow up with your partner on the results. Do not leave the office until you clearly understand what to expect. Most treatments are not cures, but they will aid in achieving and maintaining an erection and restoring your love life.

TIPS FOR TALKING

• Carefully pick a time and a quiet place. Be sure you are calm and relaxed, and have plenty of uninterrupted time.

• Listen. Repeat back to your partner what you think you heard him say. This will ensure that you really heard and understood.

• Don't judge. Never criticize or judge what your partner tells you. All feelings and concerns are valid.

• Don't get defensive. You may not like what your partner has to say, but don't argue. Acknowledge and thank him for being honest.

• Give reassurance. Tell your spouse that you love him and will be supportive during this difficult time.

YOUR ROLE IN TREATMENT

Once the doctor, your partner, and you have all agreed on a treatment, it's up to the two of you to follow instructions carefully. You may have to be patient while trying a method out for the first time, but keep trying, even if the first run-through doesn't go perfectly. Most treatments require or are enhanced by sexual stimulation, so don't forget that part.

If a treatment is not working after a fair amount of attempts and time, be sure to see the doctor and express your concerns. There are a wide variety of treatments available for ED, so if one doesn't work, select another with your doctor. Your doctor's first choice for treatment (first-line therapy) will be the simplest and easiest remedy, using an oral medication. If the first dosage isn't effective, he or she can adjust the amount of the medication or switch to another oral medication, or another treatment within the first-line therapy category. If oral medication doesn't work, your doctor will recommend a slightly more aggressive therapy: intraurethral medication or injection therapy. And remember, he or she will discuss all of this with you, since there are many options to choose from. Adjustments in dosage within the second-line therapy can also be made and tried and changed again if necessary. If the options in second-line therapy don't work, your doctor will move to the third-line therapy, which is the most aggressive form of treatment, usually requiring surgery. As you can see, there are many options within each of the three categories. Your doctor won't give up trying to find the perfect solution to a couple's problem, so you shouldn't either. Continue to encourage your partner to keep trying another treatment, even after several have failed. Correcting ED is a process you and your doctor need to work on. Treatment for ED is not always a "one time visit, follow the treatment, and everything will be okay for ever after." A treatment that works for one couple does not necessarily work for all couples. Each patient's ED is slightly different and takes the time and talent of a skilled physician and the full cooperation of the patient and his partner to resolve the problem.

YOUR ROLE IN RESTORATION OF FUNCTION

Sooner or later, and I hope sooner, you and your partner will find a suitable and satisfying treatment that will restore your sexual relationship. You may have to readjust to the new situation of a rigid penis. Be sure to see your doctor if there are any difficulties or if, in using a treatment, you are suddenly "turned off" by the mechanical aspect of the process. Remember, there are a lot of options for treating ED. You, your partner, and the doctor need to find what will work best for both of you.

YOUR PHYSICAL ROLE

Now that we've covered the male aspects of sex, let's talk a little about what is happening to *your* body as you grow older.

Your body goes through many changes as you reach midlife, possibly causing you to face some sexual dysfunction of your own. Problems with sexual desire, arousal, orgasm, and sexual pain (dyspareunia) may all occur owing to hormonal and other changes at menopause. Surgical procedures in the pelvic area can also affect the nerves and blood vessels leading to the vagina and hinder sensation for arousal. Vaginal dryness is a typical concern of many women after menopause. This common concern can be easily alleviated with over-the-counter lubricants or hormone (estrogen) replacement therapy. You should discuss any sexual problems or discomfort you have with your doctor.

Just remember that sex is for the mutual pleasure, communication, and creativity of both men and women. It is a major aspect of who we are. Be sure to share in the activity and enjoy it.

QUESTIONS MY PATIENTS' PARTNERS ASK

Q: We've been married for 18 years. It used to be real easy to make my husband have an erection when I stimulated him. Now this doesn't happen anymore. Doesn't he love me anymore? Is he seeing someone else? I'm afraid to ask him and hurt his feelings!

A: ED is very common and its occurrence increases with age. The majority of men with ED have it because of physical causes. It doesn't mean he doesn't love you or that he's having an affair. The best thing you and your husband can do is to get professional help from your doctor. Open up the line of communication warmly and supportively. Tell your husband you'll help him work through this problem.

Q: *My partner's erections are weak. He frequently is unable to enter me or complete intercourse. We talked about it but he's in complete denial that there's a problem. What should I do?*

A: Denial can happen. Reassure your partner that you love him and you're concerned about his health, not just his erections. ED is commonly associated with (and caused by) such physical conditions as high blood pressure, heart disease, and diabetes. Urge him to get evaluated and treated by a doctor. Assure him that you'll support him all the way through any treatments. Start by going with him to the doctor and staying by his side.

Q: *My partner was treated by a urologist after having ED for several years. Resuming sexual intercourse after several years of no activity has proved to be painful. Every time he penetrates me, I have a lot of pain in my vagina. I noticed that my vagina is dry. What should I do?*

A: This type of female sexual dysfunction—lack of vaginal lubrication and pain with intercourse—is common after menopause. There are some excellent over-the-counter lubricants (Astroglide or Lubrin®) that may work for you. If they don't, check with your gynecologist or a specialist in sexual dysfunction. There are some very good and effective treatments for your condition including hormones and lubricants. New treatments are under development.

IX

Restoring Sex to Your Life

> *"Relationship is not only sex, and sex is not only an erection."*

Once you've found an effective treatment for your ED (and it may take more than one try), you'll move into a new stage of awareness—your newfound sexuality. From my experience most couples have not enjoyed sex to the fullest because of ED for several years. That's a long time to miss out on a sexual relationship with your partner. And you may find that you're a little out of practice. Having successful and satisfying sex after several years of dysfunction may take a little time and some patience to achieve the level of pleasure that you remember. But it's a little like playing tennis or playing the piano: you never really forget how, but you're a bit unsteady and unsure of yourself the first time you try again. Practice and patience will soon restore your confidence and ability.

> *Several large studies have shown that the average duration of ED in patients seeking treatment for the first time is 4 years!*

No matter what treatment you have, you first have to master the mechanics of a vacuum pump, an injection needle, or an implant. Take it slowly. Practice on your own and in your doctor's office. Read and follow any instructions your doctor provides.

You may also have to work on your romancing techniques. That goes for both partners. Work on recapturing the romance, the tenderness, and the touching that filled your early courting and dating days. Some couples find that when they stop having intercourse, they also stop any fondling, caressing, or kissing. One patient of mine said, "We just stopped showing affection for each other since we were afraid to start something we couldn't finish." If that's happened to you and your partner, start rekindling the passion in your relationship by first resuming the touching, the caressing, and the kissing. Touch each other throughout the day, maybe for no special reason. Pat his arm, hold her hand, brush her cheek, give him a hug, sit close to each other while watching TV whether it's the ten o'clock news or a romantic movie, greet each other with a hug and a kiss every time you come home, and prolong your good-night kiss. You may have to work at this at first, but gradually you will become more comfortable with being physically close. After you become comfortable with general affection, participate in more erotic touching by taking a bath or shower together, applying lotion on your partner's body, or giving each other a back rub or massage. Rekindle the joy and pleasure of touching. Gradually resume caressing and fondling each other in bed. Become comfortable again with being passionate and showing affection. You're going to need to reclaim those techniques in order to eventually be successful at sexual intercourse. To use the famous baseball analogy: You might not hit a home run the first time up at bat after several years of sitting in the dugout, but you certainly don't want to strike out.

If you feel you're working at restoring the passion, but aren't making sufficient progress or haven't progressed to sexual intercourse, see your doctor. He or she may have some additional advice or suggestions, or may decide it's time for you to see a professional counselor or sex therapist. A successful sex life is possible. If you've come this far and have sought treatment, don't stop before you reach your ultimate goal: having great sex again!

Okay, so you've got the romance and foreplay under control.

Let's now talk about what to expect. If it's been a long time since you've had a rigid erection, the results of your treatment may surprise you and your partner. Your newfound virility will have restored your erection to an excellent firmness. This may be a bit off-putting to your partner, especially if she is past menopause and experiencing vaginal dryness. In order for intercourse not to be painful for her, be sure to use an over-the-counter lubricant such as Astroglide or Lubrin®.

You can restore the romance, the foreplay, and the erection, but one thing still remains a concern for many of my patients and their partners—the spontaneity of sex. At the time of writing this book, all treatments for ED require some planning and preparation for achieving an erection. For some of my patients, the loss of spontaneity is the most difficult aspect of "life after ED" to accept. They have to work at adjusting to the preplanning involved. Talk to your doctor about your need for spontaneity in making love when you are selecting the proper treatment. If your first course of treatment does not meet your needs and expectations and those of your partner, discuss another type of treatment with your doctor. New medications entering the market have different features. A long-acting medication such as Cialis™ might provide a wider window of effectiveness, thus permitting a greater scope of spontaneity. Be honest. There are many options to choose from, so keep trying new ones until you're completely satisfied.

You can certainly be spontaneous with the foreplay. Most treatments require only a brief interruption in your lovemaking. Viagra® and other oral PDE-5 inhibitors need some time to work (at least a half-hour but frequently about an hour) but that hour can easily be filled with shared activities that facilitate intimacy, such as talking, watching TV, listening to your favorite music, or dancing. Better yet, enjoy the hour in foreplay. If you try incorporating any physical process of using a vacuum device into your foreplay—much like young people include the application of a condom—that will help you feel more spontaneous.

DO'S AND DON'TS FOR RESUMING SEX

Do:

- *Be patient.*
- *Be understanding.*
- *Talk to each other about your feelings.*
- *Follow any instructions for treatment carefully and completely.*
- *Recapture the romance.*
- *Touch each other.*

Don't:

- *Get discouraged.*
- *Give up.*
- *Quit trying—call your doctor for encouragement and advice.*
- *Lose hope.*

BE SAFE

Some patients with ED might be trying to resume their sex life after a long time of having no sexual partner. The various treatments of ED are effective in restoring erectile function, but remember that they offer no protection from sexually transmitted diseases. If you feel the need to know more about this subject, ask your doctor or turn to some of the reading material in the library or on the Internet.

TIMING OF TREATMENTS AND DURATION OF RESPONSE

Viagra®: Gives you a 4- to-5-hour window for having sex, with a 1-hour lead time. That 4-hour window certainly gives you a lot of flexibility that can help you recapture some of the spontaneity of sex.

Vardenafil: Effective for about 4 to 5 hours starting about one hour after taking the pill. This also gives you flexibility and an ample window of effectiveness.

Cialis™: Will probably be effective for 24 hours and perhaps longer, so if you take the pill in the morning, you'll be ready any-time—that would be the answer to the spontaneity blues.

Uprima® or Ixense® (available in Europe): Will take effect within 10 to 25 minutes. This relatively short onset of action will meet some patients' and couples' needs for a fast effect.

With the oral medications mentioned above, it is important to understand that sexual stimulation is needed to induce the erection. The erection lasts only as long as sexual stimulation lasts. Even within the duration of effectiveness of the various medications, the erection will go away once sexual stimulation stops. Within the duration of effectiveness of a medication, it can be induced again with repeated sexual stimulation.

Injection therapy, such as Caverject®: Foreplay may need to be briefly interrupted while you inject the penis. But this treatment is effective within 5 to 15 minutes. The duration of erection is dependent upon the dose injected. Unlike oral medications, the erection induced by injection may continue even after orgasm and ejaculation and cessation of sexual stimulation. Generally, the dose is adjusted to induce an erection lasting 45 to 60 minutes.

Intraurethral therapy: Foreplay may need to be briefly interrupted while the treatment is administered. This treatment is effective within 5 to 15 minutes. In the experience of our patients, the duration of erection is variable, from 30 to 60 minutes.

Vacuum pump: This treatment interrupts foreplay. Many of my patients have said that the mechanical device destroys any natural arousal and hinders a natural experience. But if you include the vacuum device into your foreplay, like a "sex toy," you'll probably find that your perception of it as an interfering mechanical device is reduced. The erection will last as long as the rubber ring is applied. However, for safety reasons, you should not apply it for longer than half an hour.

Penile implants: This treatment is the most favored for helping with spontaneity and desire. An implant is available all the
time because it is part of your body. Preplanning for sex is almost
nonexistent. An implant is always effective and requires little ma-
nipulation. With the malleable implants the penis is always hard.
There is no limit on the duration of erection with the inflatable penile implant. You can inflate it and then deflate it any time you
want.

The whole sexual experience

It is important to understand the various domains or parts of
sexual experience. These include sexual desire, arousal/erection,
orgasm, ejaculation, and pleasure/satisfaction. Treatments of ED
are specific to the restoration of erections. They do not have a significant effect on the other domains of sexual experience, nor do
they treat other sexual dysfunctions. A patient may have ED alone
or ED plus one or more of other sexual dysfunctions, such as low
desire, difficulty with orgasm, or lack of ejaculation. With the exception of testosterone, ED treatments do not change or treat
these other sexual dysfunctions. If low desire is caused by low
testosterone, treatment with testosterone can restore sexual desire.
On the other hand, if low desire is caused by discouragement and
frustration with ED, successful treatment of ED may restore desire.

Orgasm and ejaculation should remain unchanged with the
treatment of ED. If a patient is able to have orgasm and ejaculation prior to treatment of ED, he should be able to do the same
after treatment. Similarly, if a patient has difficulty with orgasm
and ejaculation prior to treatment of ED, he may expect this to remain unchanged after treatment of ED. The other sexual dysfunctions may have specific treatments. If you have difficulty with the
other domains of your sexual experience, make sure you mention
this to your doctor and seek evaluation and treatment.

It's possible and logical to work on "rekindling the romance"

> *Restore the romance before you restore the sex.*

in your relationship while you're seeking treatment for your ED. You and your doctor *will* find an effective treatment for your problem, so at some time you'll be physically ready to resume your sex life. Be sure you and your partner are also ready emotionally.

Many patients and their partners do not consistently use or work on their treatment. They become discouraged, yearn for the "good old days" of spontaneous sex or the virility of their youth, and stop taking their medication or start using their treatment incorrectly. Experience shows that even with Viagra® there is a dropout rate of 20 to 50 percent over a period of time. Since there are no long-term studies yet available on most treatments, it is not known how many people just forget about it, lose interest, and revert to their old habits of denying themselves and their partners the joy and satisfaction of a healthy sex life.

If you should become discouraged, disillusioned, or dissatisfied with your current treatment, don't give up. See your doctor, explain the problem, and choose another treatment. Perhaps just some words of encouragement and a review of how to effectively use the treatment will help you resume your sexual activity.

QUESTIONS MY PATIENTS ASK

Q: Is it safe to have oral sex after using self-injection therapy?

A: Yes, almost all treatments of ED are compatible with various types of sexual activity. The only exception is intraurethral therapy with MUSE®. Oral sex must not be practiced when using MUSE® because the active medication alprostadil could enter your partner's mouth and throat and cause swelling and difficulty breathing.

Q: It's been 5 weeks since my surgery for an inflatable penile prosthesis. Last night, I used the implant for the first time and I had some pain with intercourse. My wife had some pain too. Is there anything wrong with my new penile implant?

A: There's probably nothing wrong with your implant. It will just take some time for you and your wife to get used to this new part of your body. You probably haven't had sex with such a hard erection for a very long time so the first few times may be a bit painful or uncomfortable. Try using a vaginal lubricant to ease your wife's discomfort.

Q: Can I have orgasm with a penile implant?

A: If you had normal orgasms before your implant, you probably won't have a problem now. A penile implant doesn't give you an orgasm or take orgasm away. It simply gives you an erect penis. It's not a treatment for those who have orgasmic difficulty.

Q: What is the filling of an inflatable penile implant?

A: It's sterile saline water. This is similar to some of the intravenous (IV) fluids commonly used in hospitals. If a leak occurs in an inflatable penile implant, the leaked fluid will get absorbed. It's not harmful.

Q: Will I be "normal" again?

A: This is a very frequently asked question. Some of my patients express the same thing as a demand: I want to be "normal" again. Doctors, especially researchers, try to shy away from the strict terms of "normal" versus "abnormal." I tell my patients, this depends to a great extent on what we mean by "normal." If normal is what one had ten, twenty or perhaps forty years ago, then it would be unrealistic to expect treatments of ED to restore all that. However, I confidently say to my patients that today we can successfully treat ED and restore satisfactory sexual function to the great majority of our patients. Many studies have repeatedly shown that treatments of ED are very successful and that patient and partner satisfaction is very high.

X

Other Issues Relating to ED

DESIRE DISORDER

One of the great triggers to having great sex is the desire for sex. You have to want sex in order to have sex. But throughout a man's life there will be various times when sexual desire ebbs and flows. This by itself is really no cause for alarm, since various psychological and social factors may contribute to low sexual desire: debilitating illness, chemotherapy, depression (which generally lessens a person's interest in almost everything, including sex), trauma, or tragedy. Medications that are prescribed to control various illnesses, or the very illnesses themselves, such as advanced stages of cancer, may have the side effect of reducing sexual desire due to fatigue and debilitation. But beyond the routine ebb and flow of life, there are some factors in a relationship that will lessen sexual desire and become cause for concern.

Partner Conflict

General unhappiness, anger, and constant quarreling over money, raising the kids, or the relatives can sabotage sexual desire in any marriage. You need a solid relationship, respect, friendship, and love to keep the sexual aspect of your marriage alive. If you can't seem to resolve your problems on your own, be sure to get some advice and guidance from a marriage counselor. Restoring your relationship will help to restore your desire.

Boredom in the Bedroom

Partners who have been together for many years may easily fall into a boring sex pattern. Same time, same place, same position, same everything equals monotonous, routine, and Boring with a capital B. Boring is a borderline lack of desire. When there's nothing exciting to look forward to, the desire to get there goes away. There really isn't a lack of desire for sex; there's just a lack of desire to do it the same old way. Changing the routine and putting the spark back into making love will also increase your desire for sex. Sex should not be a mandatory obligation or a chore like taking out the garbage. Sex should be an enjoyable experience. You may have to spark your imagination to spark up your sex life but it will be worth the effort.

Desire Discrepancy

In some relationships sexual appetites can be very different between partners: one partner has a high desire for sex and the other has a very low need. When one would love to have sex five times a week, the other would be content with five times a year. This is a problem, but usually not a medical one, unless it causes significant personal or interpersonal distress. The best way to resolve this discrepancy is to talk to a doctor, marriage counselor, or sex therapist.

Age

Some decrease in sexual desire is a natural part of aging; however, desire for sex, even if only occasional, can continue well into your seventies and eighties.

Drugs and Alcohol

Chronic drug and alcohol abuse can contribute to a low sex drive. Over time, drugs and alcohol have a toxic effect on the nervous system, damaging nerves that are critical to sexual desire and activity.

Prescription Drugs

There are prescription drugs that can cause low sexual desire. Hormonal treatment for advanced prostate cancer stops the body from producing testosterone. Drugs such as leuprolide (Lupron®) and goserilin (Zoladex®) can cause a profound decrease in sexual desire. These drugs are used in one of two ways: as a permanent, long-term treatment of metastatic (spread) prostate cancer or sometimes as a temporary treatment prior to radical prostatectomy or radiation therapy. In chronic use, low sexual desire is a permanent condition as long as the drug is taken. In such cases there currently is no effective treatment for low sexual desire. In the temporary use, normal desire will recover in 6 to 12 months after discontinuing the drug.

Hormones

The most common cause for low sexual desire is a decline in hormone levels. Healthy men require a certain amount of a variety of hormones including the most important one—testosterone—to experience a normal level of sexual desire. But as a man ages, it is expected that his sex drive eases off somewhat owing to a gradual decline in testosterone. Highest testosterone levels are found in men ages 25 to 30. The levels start to decrease around age 35, and by age 75 testosterone levels are only 50 percent of the levels of a 25-year-old. Low sexual desire can stand alone or may accompany ED.

Androgens (sex hormones) including testosterone are very important for normal sexual function. Testosterone is the main androgen secreted by males. As a man ages, his testosterone levels decline because of changes in other hormonal levels responsible for stimulating testosterone production, secretion, and protein binding. Normal levels of hormones create a body rhythm in which testosterone peaks in the morning and hits a low point in early evening. This normal rhythm ceases when there are low levels of testosterone. Men who suffer from low testosterone will experience few, if any, nighttime erections, decreased desire to masturbate, fewer sexual fantasies, decline of arousal or ED, and a low sex drive.

Treatment

It's important for your doctor to determine if you actually do have low testosterone through several blood tests before giving you any hormonal treatments. Low sexual desire can also be due to psychological or social factors in your life. Stress, illness, or a personal tragedy can cause you to have no desire for sex for some time. However, if your sex drive does not resume after the circumstances have passed, your doctor may recommend that you see a counselor to help you overcome some of the difficult situations you are currently facing.

On the other hand, if your doctor suspects that you have hypogonadism (reduced or low sex hormone levels) and confirms it with lab tests, he or she will want to start *hormone replacement therapy* (also called *androgen replacement therapy* or *testosterone replacement therapy*). Although low testosterone justifies this treatment, it is somewhat controversial for older men with borderline low testosterone, since there is uncertainty about its effectiveness and its role as related to prostate cancer. It is most appropriate for men with an abnormally low blood level of testosterone. Once hormone replacement therapy is started, you usually continue the treatment for life, since your body will stop producing natural hormones. Careful monitoring every 3 months is also required.

There are several options for testosterone therapy:

• Intramuscular (injection) therapy: Every 2 to 4 weeks your doctor will inject you with 200 mg of DEPO®-Testosterone.
• Transdermal (skin patch): A patch containing testosterone is placed on the skin daily before bedtime. Available in scrotal (Testoderm®) or nonscrotal patches (Androderm®, Testoderm-TTS®). A frequent side effect is a skin rash from the patch.
• Transdermal gel (AndroGel®): A gel containing testos-

terone that is applied to the skin once a day. This is usually very well tolerated.

Hormone treatments that are not effective are all those that are hyped on TV, the Internet, and magazines, promising you: "the virility of a 20-year-old," "super sex," "doubles your mating activity in minutes," or "sexual rejuvenating powers." Hormone creams; pills that play off the words "androgen," "testosterone," or "Viagra®"; and medications that tout themselves as "sex vitamins" are usually untested, unproven formulas that are ineffective and a waste of your money.

• Oral medication (not available in the United States): a pill is swallowed daily.

• Sublingual (not available in the United States): a pill is placed under the tongue daily.

• Implantable testosterone pellets. These pellets are implanted under the skin in a minor surgical procedure every 4 to 6 months. This form is presently available only in Europe.

If you are concerned that your sexual desire is at an all-time low, don't waste your time and money on pseudo-drugs and empty promises. See your doctor for a complete and accurate evaluation.

WAYS TO IMPROVE SEXUAL DESIRE

• Exercise.
• Watch your weight. Lose weight if you are overweight.
• Avoid heavy drinking.
• Don't take illegal drugs.
• Get treatment for depression.
• Maintain oral and physical hygiene.
• Do something to please or impress your partner.
• Work on your relationship.
• Ask your doctor for a testosterone blood test.

DIFFICULTY WITH ORGASM

An orgasm is "a pleasurable feeling (a cerebral, peripheral genital, and pelvic event) usually associated with emission and/or ejaculation." A normal sensation of orgasm requires the discharge of the tension from the orgasmic center and good coordination between the two phases of ejaculation (emission and expulsion). An orgasm does not necessarily require a rigid penis, since the nerves that control erection are different from those that control orgasm. Although orgasm and ejaculation are usually interconnected, orgasm is still possible in the absence of ejaculation (referred to as "dry orgasm"), such as after surgery for bladder or prostate cancer. In all other circumstances orgasm and ejaculation are interrelated; thus delayed orgasm also involves delayed or retarded ejaculation. There are several factors that can contribute to this problem.

• *Recreational Drugs.* A wide variety of recreational drugs can inhibit ejaculation and orgasm. Heroin, cocaine, alcohol, amphetamines, marijuana, "poppers," and methadone all are known to decrease or eliminate ejaculation and orgasm.

• *Medications.* A long list of prescribed medications can also effect the ability to reach orgasm. Antidepressants of the class known as selective serotonin reuptake inhibitors (SSRIs) such as Zoloft®, Paxil®, and Prozac® and many others can delay orgasm or completely retard ejaculation.

• *Illnesses and Injury.* Illnesses such as diabetes, Parkinson's disease, and other neurological diseases and conditions, as well as injuries to the spinal cord or pelvic area, can also affect orgasm and ejaculation.

• *Psychological Reasons.* In some cases there are psychological factors that contribute to the lack of desire or lack of arousal that is necessary for reaching orgasm.

• *Age and Hormones.* As men age, it is completely normal to experience fewer orgasms and to need intense and prolonged stimulation to achieve orgasm. This may be due to the normal decline in hormones but there have been some cases in which it is unknown why an older man can no longer achieve orgasm.

Treatments

Which treatment your doctor chooses to alleviate your delayed or retarded ejaculation and orgasm depends on the cause. If you use recreational drugs, your doctor will recommend that you discontinue using them to see if that remedies the situation. With prescribed medications, your doctor might adjust the dosage, change the prescription, or prescribe additional treatment, such as testosterone, Viagra®, or others as indicated, to solve the problem. If you're on antidepressants, you should never adjust the dosage on your own or stop taking your medication, even if you suffer from this side effect. Stopping antidepressant medications could cause your depression to recur. It is critical that you consult with your doctor.

If you have ever experienced an injury or fracture of the penis, you might require additional intense stimulation to help you achieve orgasm. With the cooperation of your partner and a sexual aid, such as a vibrator, you will be able to once again experience orgasm. If your personal concerns or circumstances, or events from your background, are inhibiting you from enjoying sexual stimulation and arousal, you would probably benefit from the advice of a sex therapist or marriage counselor to help you learn to enjoy this aspect of your life.

PEYRONIE'S DISEASE

This disease is characterized by the formation of plaque (scar tissue) in the penis, resulting in painful, curved erections that can make intercourse painfully difficult or impossible (see Figure 18). The cause of this disease is uncertain and a cure, unfortunately, is

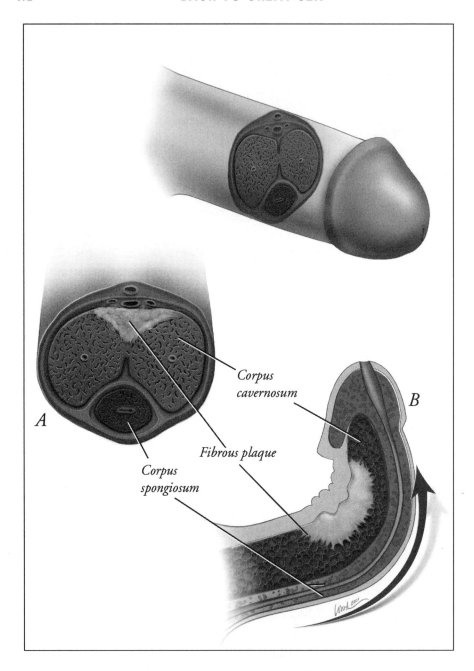

Figure 18. The anatomy of Peyronie's disease. Scar tissue (fibrosis) forms in the walls of the corpora cavernosa. This scar tissue is called plaque or fibrous plaque. The plaque is not elastic as the rest of the penis, thus causing a curvature during erection.

unknown. Sometimes this disease can be caused by trauma to the penis during intercourse due to the forceful bending of the erect penis if it hits the pubic area of the partner rather than the vaginal opening, but in most instances there is no specific cause. There are, however, various treatments that have proven effective in reducing pain and ensuring that intercourse can continue. The good news about this disease is that it occurs in only .3 to 3 percent of Caucasian men, and rarely appears in African-American men. It is most prevalent in men 45 years old and older, since the elasticity in the tissues of the penis diminishes with age. But the few men who do experience this disease are usually very concerned about it, owing to the deformity of their penis. While less than half of the men with the disease experience painful intercourse, many will experience erectile dysfunction.

Peyronie's disease is *not* caused by a sexually transmitted disease and it is *not* cancer.

> Peyronie's disease was first reported by Fallopius in 1561 but made popular in 1743 by François Gigot de la Peyronie, a surgeon to King Louis XV of France. The disease has since been known by his name. Dr. Peyronie recommended use of Barege spa water and mercurial ointments to treat the disease. In the 1800s iodine, arsenic, and camphor were used. Peyronie's disease has a colorful history and much has been written about it, but a cure for it has yet to be found.

The symptoms for this disease will evolve slowly—with a gradual curving of the penis during erection. Symptoms may include:

• Curvature of the penis during erection (may interfere with sexual intercourse)
• Pain during erection
• The penis appears shorter and/or narrower

- A hard area on the top (most common) or bottom side of the penis can be felt
- Erectile dysfunction

At the start of the disease you will probably experience a painful period of inflammation. The pain isn't usually severe, but it may interfere with your sexual function until the inflammation ceases. Intercourse may be difficult owing to pain, curvature of the penis, and lack of rigidity. As the disease progresses, your penis may become progressively more curved over a period of a year. Once the scar tissue has matured, however, the curving stops and doesn't get any worse.

Treatments for Peyronie's disease range from a "wait and see" stance to surgery. Your doctor will need to discuss with you what will be the best form of treatment for your individual situation. Seeking early evaluation and treatment is the best option for reducing pain and limiting the progression of the disease. Your doctor's goal in treating the disease will be to prescribe methods that seem to help in order to keep you sexually active. As of now, there is no known cure for this disease except for surgery to correct the curvature.

"Wait and See"

Sometimes all that you'll need is education: awareness of what is happening and information about the disease, what your options are, and what to expect. If the curvature of your penis is mild and you can still have intercourse, most doctors prefer to do nothing beyond relaying information and giving encouragement. Believe it or not, sometimes this disease improves all by itself—disappearing as mysteriously as it first appeared.

Oral Medications

A variety of oral treatments have been tried over the years with varying results. At this time no one, oral treatment is universally supported by doctors since there is a lack of controlled scientific studies.

Your doctor may prescribe a dose of 800 to 1000 units daily of *Vitamin E* to control the early course of the disease. Vitamin E is inexpensive and free of any side effects, so it is frequently used even during a "wait and see" stage. *Potaba*® may be prescribed (12 mg daily) to reduce plaque size and penile deformity. This medication is not very successful and its side effects include frequent upset stomach. *Colchicine* (0.6 mg 3 times a day) is another oral therapy. This medication was originally used for the treatment of an unrelated condition, gout. But it has been found to be effective in improving pain and deformity at the early stage of Peyronie's disease.

Injection Therapy

Various drugs have been injected directly into the plaque (scar tissue) in the penis to "dissolve" it. Researchers have been studying a variety of drugs (orgotein, steroids—not recommended—verapamil, interferon, and collagenase) with varying results but all need additional study.

Currently, early results of *verapamil* injections and creams are encouraging. In one study this drug decreased or softened plaque, or decreased the curvature of the penis in patients with the disease. This drug is not approved by the FDA for use in Peyronie's disease and its use for treating the disease is still considered off-label. However, results from studies suggest that it may be a reasonable approach in select patients for treatment when the plaque is noncalcified and the penile curvature is less than 30 degrees.

Another injection drug being explored is *interferon*. In one study where this investigational drug was injected biweekly into the plaque, the patients reported softening of the plaque, absence of penile pain, improved curvature, and a decrease in plaque size.

Iontophoresis

In the search for finding a treatment that is less invasive than injection therapy, several doctors are now testing a new method of delivering drugs into the plaque with an electrical current. This treatment, called *iontophoresis,* uses a mixture of two (verapamil and dexaethasone) or three (dexaethasone, lidocaine, and verapamil) drugs that are administered with an electrical current. Patients in various studies have reported a decrease in pain, decrease in plaque size, improvement in curvature of the penis, and improved sexual function.

If you have ED along with Peyronie's disease, one of the various treatments for ED may be effective and recommended by your doctor.

Surgical Treatments

Surgery, the only known correction for Peyronie's disease, must be carefully considered before being selected.

Patients who qualify for surgery:

- Have had the disease for at least 1 year or longer.
- Have a curvature that exceeds 30 degrees, interfering with sexual intercourse.
- Have a curvature that has stopped progressing for at least 3 months prior to surgery.
- Do not have continuing pain.

In the past few years, old surgical techniques have been modified and new surgical techniques have been developed that are less aggressive. The goal is to reduce the complications of erectile dysfunction, penile sensory loss, and penile deformity. One option for surgery, if you are not experiencing erectile problems, is for your doctor to cut the plaque or scar tissue in the penis and insert a graft (venous patch graft from a vein in the leg). This procedure is effective in 70 to 80 percent of patients.

A second option is for your surgeon to shorten the opposite side of the penis to eliminate the curvature. This results in a somewhat shorter penis, but does restore the ability for sexual intercourse.

A third option, most frequently used for those individuals who also suffer from ED and do not respond to other ED treatments, is to implant a prosthesis into the penis. The implant straightens the penis and gives you dependable erections for the rest of your life.

Peyronie's disease, although still a mystery as to cause and cure, continues to receive attention from the medical profession. A wide variety of treatments are being studied in order for doctors to manage the illness and provide a cure. Until a certain treatment is agreed upon, doctors recommend that their patients not ignore the symptoms, but seek professional help in the first or second month of the disease in order for any treatment to be the most effective.

PREMATURE EJACULATION

Premature ejaculation is defined as the inability to control the rapid expulsion of seminal fluid. Ejaculation takes place too quickly and occurs before, or soon after (less than one minute) penetration of the vagina. Some therapists describe ejaculation as premature if you are unable to continue intercourse for more than 1 minute without ejaculating, while others believe that you should be able to satisfy your partner more than 50 percent of the time. Premature ejaculation is a common physical condition, occurring in 25 to 40 percent of all adult men. It can prevent or undermine stable relationships and marriage, and can lead to depression, anxiety, personality disorders, and other more serious sexual dysfunction. Masters and Johnson, the renowned sex scientists, stated that premature ejaculation is the most frequent male sexual dysfunction, but men typically do not seek treatment because they consider it futile or are told that there is no valid medical therapy.

Premature ejaculation is defined as:

Persistent or recurrent ejaculation with minimal stimulation before, on, or shortly after penetration, and before the person wishes it. Age, novelty of the sexual partner or situation, and recent frequency of sexual activity are taken into consideration.

The disturbance causes marked distress or interpersonal difficulty.

The premature ejaculation is not due exclusively to the direct effects of a substance (e.g., withdrawal from opiates).

—American Psychiatric Association's Diagnostic and Statistical Manual, *IV 1994.*

Causes

For many years physicians assumed that primary (lifelong) premature ejaculation was psychological and caused by anxiety regarding unresolved fears of the vagina, conflicts with a particular partner, anger and hostility toward women, or a bad habit learned from early, hurried sexual experiences. Secondary (acquired after a period of normal ejaculation) premature ejaculation could be caused by ED since a man conditions himself to climax quickly before he loses his erection.

Only in a small number of patients is a cause known. The majority of cases are considered idiopathic (the cause is unknown). Think of the process of ejaculation as an alarm clock. If your alarm clock rings too early, you don't say the alarm clock is broken—you just figure it was set for too early a time. It's the same with ejaculation. Premature or early ejaculation doesn't mean something is wrong; it just means that the timing is too early. Behavioral modification in sex therapy helps to "reset the clock" of the timing in ejaculation.

There is now evidence that premature ejaculation could be a physical problem. Trauma to the nervous system, pelvic fractures, diseases of the urinary tract and prostate gland, as well as heart disease, diabetes, hardening of the arteries, and withdrawal from alcoholism or drug abuse may all be physical causes for this dysfunction.

Treatments

Behavior Modification

For many years the only course of treatment was sexual behavior modification. Behavior modification is widely used today and can be helpful. The goal of this therapy is to overcome any fears of sexual performance and replace them with productive thoughts of ejaculatory control, and reaffirm the role of intimacy in lovemaking. This therapy encourages the man to become more familiar with the feelings and sensations leading up to orgasm so he can gain better control of ejaculation. Since the early 1970s therapists have suggested several techniques to achieve this control: self-stimulation exercises; the stop-start, squeeze technique; progressive sensate focus exercises; and the "quiet vagina" technique.

Behavioral treatment usually begins with the man alone engaging in a *self-stimulation* exercise in which he brings himself to a midrange level of excitement before pausing. After repeating this several times he is then permitted to ejaculate. The purpose of this exercise is to help him experience a midlevel of excitement and slow down his arousal, thus slowing down ejaculation.

The next level of exercise includes the partner stimulating the man repeatedly to a high level of excitement either orally or manually (and later vaginally) but stopping prior to ejaculation. This *"stop-start" procedure* allows the man's arousal to decrease and thus delay orgasm. After repeating this exercise several times, the man is permitted to ejaculate. A variation of this technique is for the partner to quickly but firmly *squeeze* the man's glans penis after stopping stimulation to lower his arousal. The squeeze can result in a partial loss of erection, however.

Sensate focus exercises help the man develop an awareness of his arousal level through nonsexual stimulation. In a slow, gradual fashion the man and his partner take turns giving and receiving pleasure through touching one another (nongenital, nonbreast stimulation). As the man gains ejaculation control, these areas are included in the exercise.

"*Quiet vagina*" is another variation of the stop-start technique that includes intercourse. After successfully stimulating the man manually, the woman sits astride or lies on top of the man and, without any thrusting or rhythmic movement, envelops his penis in her vagina. The purpose of this is to desensitize the man to the warm environment of the vagina. After the man masters the "quiet vagina" for a long period of time, the woman introduces slow movement. The man asks her to stop when he is excited and the couple then quietly sits or lies together until the man's arousal decreases. Then the movement is repeated again. After several repetitions of this exercise, the man eventually is allowed to ejaculate.

These techniques require the cooperation and understanding of the couple to be successful. At times the female partner may feel used and unimportant, but it is important for her to focus on the ultimate goal—increased pleasurable sex for both her and her partner. Unfortunately a three-year follow-up study evaluating treatment and assessing long-term benefits of these techniques found that 75 percent of the patients showed no signs of lasting improvement.

Drug Therapy

Doctors and researchers have been investigating several drugs that have a side effect of delaying or impairing ejaculation. They have rationalized that a drug that delays ejaculation from "normal" to "impaired" may be effective in delaying "premature" to "normal." Although none of these drugs is currently approved by the FDA for the treatment of premature ejaculation, the use of antidepressants for managing this condition has been explored by a few physicians.

• Application of a *local anaesthetic gel* for 30 minutes prior to intercourse has shown good results. It is necessary, however, to thoroughly wash off the gel before intercourse or the partner will also be affected by the drug.

• *Clomipramine (Anafranil®)*, a tricyclic antidepressant (25 mg taken 12 to 24 hours before intercourse) has been effective in controlled studies in delaying ejaculation and enhancing sexual enjoyment; however, the side effects are not pleasant: sleepiness, weight gain, difficulty in swallowing, and making ED worse.

• *Fluoxetine (Prozac®)*, taken in a dose of 10 mg daily for a week and 20 mg daily thereafter, proved effective for delaying ejaculation after 4 weeks of treatment.

• *Paroxetine HC1 (Paxil®)*, taken in doses of 20 to 40 mg daily, has also been effective and safe for the treatment of premature ejaculation in several studies.

• *Sertralin (Zoloft®)* is similar to Prozac® at doses of 50 to 100 mg.

New medications for the treatment of premature ejaculation are currently being researched. The use of the abovementioned medications for premature ejaculation is considered off-label. Some doctors are concerned that treating premature ejaculation with a prescription drug will not be in the best interest of the patient and his partner. They point out that the couple may really need to resolve some personal or psychological problems as well as the dysfunction in order to assure a fulfilling sex life. Fixing a sexual problem such as premature ejaculation will not fix any nonsexual problems you are also having in your relationship. Counseling and therapy can be very beneficial in that regard. Future research and additional understanding of premature ejaculation will probably blend the physical and psychological aspects of this sexual problem.

QUESTIONS MY PATIENTS ASK

Q: I seem to have lost all sexual feelings. Things that used to arouse me, like movies or advertisements, have no effect on me at all. What's wrong?

A: There may be multiple reasons for your lack of desire that you should take a look at. You may need to put a little "zip" into your relationship if you have a long-term partner. Boredom and routine in the bedroom can hinder desire. You may have a medical problem of low hormone levels but you need to review this with your doctor (don't succumb to the temptation of buying "mail-order" creams or pills that promise to increase your sex drive—they're a waste of money). You could also be depressed or your low sexual desire is a side effect of ED. If the minor adjustments aren't effective, make an appointment with your doctor to find out if there is an underlying medical concern.

Q: Recently my wife stopped using the pill and I've started using a condom. Suddenly I'm having problems reaching orgasm. What could be wrong?

A: I'll assume that you have mutually chosen to change your method of birth control and are using condoms as an intermediate step until you want to conceive. If that's the case, your condom may be your problem. It might not be allowing you the stimulation you need to reach orgasm, or it may be too tight or its quality may be poor. Try a different type of condom (or several). If your problem continues, talk to your doctor.

Q: What are aphrodisiacs?

A: Aphrodisiacs are certain foods, herbal drugs, or nutritional supplements that some people claim increase sexual desire (libido) or enhance erections and orgasm. Almost all of these substances have not been through rigorous scientific research to prove their effectiveness and safety. Therefore, the claims are not valid.

The word "aphrodisiac" comes from the name "Aphrodite," the ancient Greek goddess of love and beauty.

Q: What is the cause of premature ejaculation?

A: The majority of men with premature or rapid ejaculation have this condition all of their sexually active lives. It's thought by most researchers that this is a behavioral condition.

Q: Recently I started having difficulty reaching orgasm. What could cause this?

A: Difficulty in reaching orgasm is referred to as retarded orgasm. Some men (especially older men) have this problem. For no clear reason, they require intense and prolonged stimulation to reach orgasm. A common cause of retarded orgasm is the use of antidepressants such as Prozac®, Zoloft® and Paxil®. These medications, called selective serotonin reuptake inhibitors (SSRIs), are known to delay orgasm as a side effect. Other causes of retarded orgasm include neuropathy secondary to diabetes, alcoholism, and pelvic trauma.

Q: What exactly is Peyronie's disease?

A: Peyronie's disease is the formation of fibrosis (scar tissue) in the penis. The tissues of the penis are supposed to be elastic so they expand during erection. Scar tissue is not elastic. Therefore it causes curvature and other penile shape deformities.

Q: Does Peyronie's disease always need surgery?

A: No, in approximately half of all cases the condition either improved spontaneously or stabilized with minimal sexual disability. Only cases that persist with severe penile curvature interfering with intercourse require surgery.

XI

Choosing a Physician, Facility, and Treatment

The issue of privacy is certainly an important one, especially when it involves so personal a matter as your sex life. Everyone desires and deserves as much privacy as they feel is necessary. Whether you are a well-known personality in your community, a high-profile political leader, a famous actor or singer, or a private person who has no desire to have neighbors, friends, and casual acquaintances know about your seeking help for your sexual difficulty, you deserve to be protected from any embarrassing encounters. If you are seeking help from your primary care physician, you will pretty much remain anonymous. No one really knows why you are visiting your doctor—it could be for a flu shot. Even a visit to a specialist, such as a urologist, does not necessarily imply you have a sexual problem. Urologists see men, women, and children for all types of treatments. However, if your urologist is particularly well known for the treatment of ED, being spotted in his or her waiting room could suggest what your problem is. But remember, if the other person is there, each of you can guess why the other is seeking help.

If privacy is a requirement for you, your specialist will probably be very sensitive to your needs. Many specialists reserve the first and last appointments of the day for "high-profile" individuals who are well-known public figures with familiar faces through

TV or other media or those seeking privacy. In extreme cases, where privacy is of the utmost importance (for example, for a celebrity), a doctor may arrange for an "after-hours" appointment to ensure that no other patients are around and there is very little chance of being recognized. Most doctors are also willing to contact you in whatever way you are most comfortable with: at home, or not at home; at the office only or never at your work; at a post office box, or through e-mail or voice mail. Be specific in sharing your needs for privacy. Your doctor's nurses and assistants should be aware that your problem needs to be addressed in the strictest confidence.

> *Privacy in treating ED is important to men worldwide. In fact, owing to the lack of privacy, many men in certain countries do not seek treatment for their ED. Although Viagra® was approved in many countries to treat ED after it received FDA approval in the United States, some men do not ask for a prescription for the drug. The problem of ED in some cultures and countries goes untreated because of the lack of privacy, embarrassment and the social stigma and taboo attached to this problem. Few men will even admit to having ED because it is such a private issue. Some men might travel to a different geographic location, where they will have complete privacy in receiving a prescription for Viagra® or another treatment.*

CHOOSING A PHYSICIAN

Family Doctor/Primary Care Physician/Internist

Usually the first doctor you seek help and advice from for treating your ED will be the doctor you see on a routine or annual basis for your physical, flu shot, rashes, infections, and persistent coughs or colds. You can easily approach the subject of ED during a routine physical; however, it's better if you make a dedicated appointment about this particular problem. If you find it difficult to make the appointment, tell the nurse: "I'd like to see the doctor to talk about a personal health problem I'm having."

Be prepared to discuss the exact nature of your problem. The more specific you can be, the faster your doctor can provide the ideal treatment for you. You should also review and fill out the "ED Individual Needs Questionnaire" on page 191 and the "Comprehensive Questionnaire and Data Form" on page 207 before seeing your doctor. If you find that your primary doctor is uncomfortable talking to you about ED, ask for a referral to a specialist. Your doctor may also recommend that you see a specialist, depending on your particular situation.

Remember, you have as much right to ask for medical help for ED as you do for any other health problem. If one doctor does not take your problem seriously, seek help from another physician.

Urologist

A urologist is a specialist who treats diseases of the genitals and urinary tract. He or she is the doctor who most frequently treats ED, especially in those patients who have a physical cause to their problem. Urologists provide routine evaluation and treatment as well as perform special tests to evaluate the function of the nerves, arteries, and veins that control an erection. They also prescribe medications and perform surgery to correct ED problems.

Psychologists/Psychiatrists

These specialists treat the psychological and relational causes of ED—depression, anxiety, sexual inhibition, and problems with self-image and self-esteem. Your doctor might recommend that you seek the services of one of these professionals while taking medication or using another treatment for ED. ED treatments can be far more effective if used in tandem with counseling.

Sex Therapists and Marriage Counselors

These mental health professionals work with individuals and couples who need guidance and instruction in sexual knowledge and techniques as well as partner relationships and communication. They frequently recommend exercises and behavior modifications to practice at home. Most individuals are highly satisfied with the help they receive from these professionals. This type of treatment is cost-effective, short-term, and very much results-oriented.

Endocrinologist

An endocrinologist may be the specialist your doctor sends you to if your ED is due to a hormonal problem, such as a low testosterone level, a pituitary gland problem, or a thyroid disorder.

There are a wide variety of treatments and specialists who are available to help you treat your ED. If the first treatment prescribed is not as effective as you had hoped, be sure to see your doctor again and explain the problem. There are many more treatments that you can try, if you are willing to work with your doctor on the problem. Doctors follow a step-care model that offers first-, second-, and third-line treatments for ED. (See Table 1, page 69.) For some men, the first treatment may be adequate; for others it may require several dose changes, a variety of different treatments, or surgery; but 99 percent of men with ED can find a suitable and acceptable treatment to regain their sexual well-being and get them back to great sex, if they are open-minded, willing to follow instructions, and follow up with their doctor.

Check the Resources at the back of this book to help locate an appropriate physician or counselor.

CHOOSING A FACILITY

Private Practice (Individual or Group)

This is the most common type of practice for a primary care doctor or a specialist. Check your insurance plan to see if you need a referral from your primary care physician before seeing a specialist. Your primary care doctor may be the best and first step for seeking help.

Sexual Dysfunction Centers

These types of centers usually exist in big cities. They are commonly associated with the department of urology of a major university's medical school or hospital. A sexual dysfunction center can provide you with advanced expertise in this subspecialty and refer you as well to other specialists such as psychiatrists and sex therapists if that is also needed. A university center will also be able to take advantage of the many resources available from the university.

Other types of services are available through a urology clinic of a Veterans Administration hospital, the Armed Forces medical services, and municipal clinics.

CHOOSING THE BEST TREATMENT

Finding and choosing the best treatment requires an open mind, a willingness to listen to all the options, and continuous communication and follow-up with your doctor. In general, you and your doctor will review each treatment and choose the one that best fits the following criteria:

- Simple to use
- Noninvasive (doesn't require surgery or an incision)
- Painless
- High success rate
- Brings your sex life closest to naturalness and spontaneity
- Few minor, short-lasting side effects
- Affordable
- Satisfactory to your individual needs
- Satisfactory to you and your partner as a couple

CHOOSING A TREATMENT

Selecting a treatment is a very personal decision that needs to reflect your and your partner's preferences. Here are some questions to think about—and ask your doctor:

- *How effective and safe is the treatment?*
- *How does my partner feel about the treatment?*
- *Is it convenient and comfortable to use?*
- *Does it fit with my lifestyle?*
- *How much does the treatment cost? Will my insurance pay for some or all of it?*

As an example, let's discuss the choice of a penile implant after failure of other medical treatments. If you, your partner, and your doctor agree that a penile implant is the best option of treatment for you, then you will have to make some additional decisions. Your first choice will have to be between the malleable rod implant or an inflatable implant. Ask your doctor to let you see and touch the various implants before your surgery. Practice using them to find out which of them you are most comfortable with or are the easiest for you to use. You may find that the malleable rod is best for you to use if you have any physical limitations: vision problems, blindness, weakness in your hands, tremors from Parkinson's disease, or paralysis. The inflatable implant requires good eye–hand coordination and manual dexterity. If you have limitations in those areas but still prefer the inflatable implant, you may consider this option if your partner is willing to inflate and deflate the implant for you. The malleable rod is simple to use. The inflatable implant is a bit more complicated but gives the penis a more natural feel and appearance and is much preferred by most patients.

If you make the choice for an inflatable implant, you will then have to choose among a one-, two-, or three-piece model. In this decision your surgeon will have the ability and experience to make the choice for you. Many doctors have a strong preference for one style over another, so they will be able to advise you. Surgery for the one- and two-piece is simpler, but the three-piece implant is the "top of the line" of implants and gives the most patient–partner satisfaction.

This last point—"Does it satisfy my individual needs"—may require you to give some thought to exactly what those needs and desires are. The "ED Individual Needs Questionnaire," below, lists questions I frequently ask my patients to help them evaluate their desires and needs, as well as those of their partner.

ED INDIVIDUAL NEEDS QUESTIONNAIRE

Review the questions. Circle your answers and communicate the results to your doctor. There are no right or wrong answers. Feel free to add comments if one of the suggested answers doesn't really express how you or your partner feels.

1. How important is sexual function to you?
   a. Extremely important. I can't live without sex.
   b. Somewhat important.
   c. Not important. If I can't regain my function through a simple and easy process, forget it.

2. How important is your sexual function/ability to your partner?
   a. Extremely important. Our relationship will be over if I don't do something.
   b. Somewhat important. Sex would be nice, but our relationship will survive without it.
   c. Not important. Sex is not important in our relationship. It will survive without sex. Intercourse doesn't matter to my partner.

3. How determined are you to regain erectile function?
  a. Very determined. I'll try anything.
  b. Somewhat determined. I'll only try certain treatments.
  c. Not determined. I'll only try what's easy and convenient; otherwise forget it.

4. How patient are you?
  a. Very patient. I'm very persistent and will work at something until I have it right.
  b. Somewhat patient. I'll give it more than one or two tries, then I get doubtful.
  c. Impatient. I'll try something once, but usually do not spend much time if I don't master it quickly.

5. How understanding and willing is your partner?
  a. Very. My partner is determined to work this out with me.
  b. Somewhat. We'll try anything once or twice together, but we expect results.
  c. Not understanding. My partner believes this is *my* problem, not our problem.

6. Have you talked openly with your partner about your problem?
      yes   no

7. How long have you been in your present relationship?
  a. Less than 1 year
  b. 1–10 years
  c. 11–25 years
  d. over 25 years

8. How old are you? ___ years

9. How old is your partner? ___ years

10. Are you willing to consider:

a. Oral medication	yes	no
b. Mechanical devices	yes	no
c. Injections	yes	no
d. Urethral therapy	yes	no
e. Creams or gels	yes	no
f. Implant	yes	no

11. Is your partner willing to work with you on:

a. Oral medication	yes	no
b. Mechanical devices	yes	no
c. Injections	yes	no
d. Urethral therapy	yes	no
e. Creams or gels	yes	no
f. Implant	yes	no

Honest and open communication with your doctor will provide him or her with a better understanding of your personality, your partner, and your overall relationship. For any treatment to be successful, you and your partner need to follow instructions carefully, openly discuss any concerns or problems with your doctor, and be patient with one another as well as with any requirements of the treatment.

You can succeed. You can restore your sexual well-being, resume a high quality of life, and enjoy great sex once again.

TABLE 3

Treatment Chart

TREATMENT	ADVANTAGES	DISADVANTAGES	COST
Oral medications	On-demand use. Easy to use. Effective. Safe.	Takes time to work. Limited: one pill per day. Minor side effects.	$10 per pill. Insurance coverage variable according to individual policy.
Vacuum constriction device	Gives immediate results. Requires no surgery. Is drug-free. No serious side effects.	Cumbersome. A mechanical device that interrupts foreplay. Can cause pain, lack of ejaculation, bruising. Penis appears bluish and may be cool.	$140–$500 (one-time fee). Covered by some insurance companies.
Counseling/ sex therapy	Noninvasive. Anyone can use. Increases effectiveness of other treatments.	Uncertain effectiveness. Dependent on you and your partner's motivation. Can be expensive.	$50–300 per hour. Not covered by insurance.
Intraurethral drug therapy	On-demand use. Can use twice in 24 hours. Easy to use. Relatively safe. Relatively effective.	Invasive local administration. Side effect: pain. Oral sex prohibited. Interrupts foreplay.	$18–$25 per use. Covered by most insurance companies.
Intracavernosal injection therapy	On-demand use. Highly effective. Safe. Nonsurgical. Short onset of action.	Limited use: 3 times per week. Invasive local administration. Side effects: pain, priapism, scarring. Interrupts foreplay.	$25 per use. Covered by most insurance companies.
Penile implant	Long-term remedy. Immediately effective. No limits of frequency of use. High satisfaction by users and partners.	Surgery required. Possible mechanical failure. Length and girth of penis may be altered.	$8,000–$15,000. Covered by insurance.
Hormone replacement therapy	Improves sex drive, sex function, energy, and mood. Nonsurgical.	Once needed, must continue for life. Periodic evaluation of prostate required.	$170–$180 per month (gel). $9–$20 per month (injections).

The above cost figures are estimates only. They may vary with time and location.

Afterword

Preventing ED

If you are reading this book, you're already concerned and suspect that you have some degree of ED. And since ED is a progressive condition, it will only get worse, not better, if you leave it alone. So now you're probably asking: "Was there anything I could have done to prevent myself from getting ED?" or "What did I do wrong?"

Well, you probably didn't do anything wrong. Getting older is not a right or wrong situation that you have any control over. However, there are several things you can do to delay the onset of ED as long as possible. Or if you have mild ED, these same modifications to your lifestyle can slow down and control the progressive nature of ED from moving into the moderate and advanced stages.

1. Exercise. A sedentary lifestyle is not good for your general health or your sexual health. Walk or work out at least three times a week for 30 minutes each session.
2. If you are a diabetic, keep good control of your diabetes: Follow your diet instructions, control your weight, take your diabetes medication, exercise, and control your blood sugar.
3. Don't smoke. And if you do smoke, stop as soon as possible.
4. Don't drink too much alcohol.
5. Have sex regularly. Exercise your penis. There are strong

indications that the penis loses function if it is not used
regularly. "Use it or lose it."

6. Don't take illegal recreational drugs. They can damage
   your nervous system, and you need healthy nerves for
   good sexual function.
7. Get a yearly physical to maintain your general health and
   reveal any disease for early treatment and control.
8. Avoid fatty foods and watch your weight.
9. Have your cholesterol checked: men with high cholesterol risk getting ED.
10. Stay happy. Depression, stress, and anger can affect your
    sex life.
11. Lead a balanced life. Keep your work, family, civic, and
    religious responsibilities in balance so you have some
    time left for yourself, for leisure and exercise.
12. If you choose biking as your form of exercise, be sure to
    use padded bike shorts or a gel-filled bike seat. Padding
    will protect you from injuring the critical nerves and ar-
    teries that must remain healthy to produce an erection.
    Avoid excessive mountain biking with uneven and rough
    terrain that can cause injuries from hitting the crossbar of
    the bike.

In brief: If you want a good sex life, make time for it, and in-
vest in your general health.

Glossary

ADAM: Androgen Decline in the Aging Male, also known as andropause or male menopause.

Anatomy: the study of the human body.

AndroGel®: The brand name of the drug testosterone used as a gel therapy through the skin for the treatment of testosterone deficiency, hypogonadism, or andropause (ADAM).

Androgen: male sexual hormone. There are several androgens. The main one is testosterone.

Andropause: male menopause; decline in male sexual hormones in the aging male.

Anejaculation: absence of ejaculation.

Anorgasmia: inability to achieve orgasm.

Arteriosclerosis: hardening of the arteries.

Atherosclerosis: The vascular disease caused by fat deposits into the walls of blood vessels, thus creating risk of clogging, obstruction and complications such as heart attack, stroke, weak circulation in the legs, and ED.

Caverject®: the brand name of the injectable drug prostaglandin E_1 or alprostadil used for the treatment of ED.

Cavernosometry: a test to measure the venous leak and the pressure in the penis during an artificially induced erection with medications and infusion of saline

Cavernosography: a test using a dye injected into the penis to examine via x-ray a venous leak in the penis.

Cialis™: the brand name of the oral drug Tadalafil (IC_{351}) used for the treatment of ED.

Corpora cavernosa: the cylindrical-shaped structures inside the penis that contain the erectile tissue.

Delayed ejaculation: undue delay in reaching ejaculation in spite of adequate and continuing sexual stimulation.

Dyspareunia: pain during sexual intercourse.

Ejaculation: passage of seminal fluid through the urethra and its expulsion from the penis.

Emission: the transfer of sperm cells from the testicles to the urethra through the vasa.

Endocrinologist: a doctor specializing in disorders of hormones.

Erectile dysfunction (frequently abbreviated as ED): the consistent or recurrent inability of a man to attain and/or maintain a penile erection sufficient for sexual performance.

Erection: "hard-on," a rigid penis.

Fibrosis: scarring or scar tissue.

Flaccid: soft or limp.

Glans penis: the head of the penis.

Hypertension: high blood pressure.

Impotence: a general term used most frequently to describe ED, but also may refer to various sexual dysfunctions: loss of libido, orgasmic or ejaculatory problems, or erection difficulties. The National Institutes of Health recommends the replacement of this term with the more accurate one: erectile dysfunction (ED).

Libido: sex drive, desire for sexual activity.

MUSE®: Medicated Urethral System for Erection; an intraurethral therapy using the drug prostaglandin E_1 or alprostadil.

Neuropathy: nerve damage.

NPTR test: nocturnal penile tumescence and rigidity test; a test taken on an ambulatory basis using the RigiScan to measure girth and rigidity of the penis during sleep erections.

Organic: physical.

Orgasm: a pleasurable feeling usually associated with emission and/or ejaculation.

PDE-5 inhibitors: Phospho diesterase type-5 inhibitors. This is a class of oral medications used for the treatment of ED. This class includes currently: Viagra®, Cialis™ and Vardenafil. Other medications are in various stages of development. Generally, this class of medications has proven to be highly effective and well tolerated.

Performance anxiety: a fear of not being able to have sexual relations triggered by memories of past failures.

Perineum: the area including the penis and the anus.

Premature ejaculation: the occurrence of ejaculation before or soon after the beginning of intercourse.

Priapism: a prolonged, painful erection that lasts more than 4 hours continuously.

Prosthesis: an artificial replacement for a missing body part.

Radical prostatectomy: a surgical procedure to remove the entire prostate, as well as the seminal vesicles and some lymph nodes.

Retrograde ejaculation: the backward passage of semen into the bladder after emission, causing sperm to appear in the urine.

Rigid: firm and erect, in reference to the penis; a "hard-on."

RigiScan®: a device that performs ambulatory testing of nocturnal erections.

Sex therapist: a specialist (frequently a psychologist) specializing in psychological or behavioral therapy of sexual dysfunctions.

Testosterone: the main male sex hormone.

Uprima® or Ixense®: brand names depending on the geographic location of the sublingual tablet of apomorphine used for the treatment of ED.

Urethra: the urinary channel in the penis.

Urologist: a doctor specializing in treating diseases of the genitals and urinary tract.

Vardenafil: The brand name of the oral drug Vardenafil used for the treatment of ED.

Vascular: referring to blood vessels, such as arteries, veins, and capillaries.

Vasoconstriction: closing or narrowing of the blood vessels caused by the contraction of the smooth muscle cells in the penis to cause flaccidity.

Vasodilation: opening or widening of the blood vessels caused by the relaxation of the smooth muscle cells in the penis to cause an erection.

VCD: vacuum constriction device used to create an erection; a vacuum pump.

Venous leak: a problem in which the blood leaks out of the penis back into the general circulation, so that an erection is not maintained for very long.

Viagra®: the brand name for the oral drug sildenafil citrate used for the treatment of ED.

Resources

American Urological Association (AUA)
1120 North Charles Street
Baltimore, MD 21201-5559
(410) 727-1100
Web site: www.auanet.org

The AUA is a nonprofit organization that represents urologists and scientists in the field of urology. This association promotes the highest standards of urological care, research, education, and formulation of healthcare policy. The AUA can help you find a urologist in your area.

American Association of Sex Educators, Counselors and Therapists (AASECT)
PO Box 238
Mount Vernon, IA 52314
Web site: www.aasect.org

This organization represents a variety of health professionals who are advocates of understanding human sexuality and healthy sexual behavior. AASECT can help you find a counselor or therapist in your area.

American Association for Marriage and Family Therapy (AAMFT)
1133 15th Street, Northwest

Suite 300
Washington, DC 20005-2710
(202) 223-2329
Web site: www.aamft.org

This organization represents marriage and family therapists, who treat a wide variety of mental health disorders, including marital stress and relationship problems. Therapists also can work with doctors when medical treatment is needed. The AAMFT can help you locate a therapist in your area.

American Diabetes Association, Inc.
National Office
1701 North Beauregard Street
Alexandria, VA 22311
(800) DIABETES
Web site: www.diabetes.org

This leading nonprofit health organization provides diabetes research, information, and advocacy. It offers free publications for people with diabetes, including several brochures and articles on diabetes in general. The ADA also can help you find a doctor who specializes in diabetes in your area. Check in your phone book for a local chapter.

The National Institute of Diabetes, Digestive and Kidney Diseases (NIDDK)
Web site: www.niddk.nih.gov
Or: www.niddk.nih.gov/health/urolog/pubs/impotnce/impotnce.htm

This research institute is part of the National Institutes of Health (NIH), and conducts and supports research on ED and other serious diseases. Its Web site offers information on impotence and provides links to other government Web sites with information on sexuality, health, and clinical research.

National Kidney and Urologic Diseases Information Clearinghouse
3 Information Way
Bethesda, MD 20892-3580
Web site: www.nkudic@info.niddk.nih.gov

You can order publications on kidney and urologic diseases from
this clearinghouse using the above address or e-mail.

World Health Organization (WHO)
Web site: www.who.dk.

This organization in conjunction with the International Society
for Impotence Research held the 1st International Consultation
on Erectile Dysfunction on July 1–3, 1999 in Paris, France. This
gathering of over 150 recognized, international experts in the field
of ED resulted in a major textbook called *Erectile Dysfunction*.
This book is a valuable working tool for all those involved in the
diagnosis and treatment of ED.

WebMD
www.webmd.com

This is an online health information source that helps consumers,
physicians, and other providers. Consumers can access health
news, articles, research reports, etc.

OTHER WEB SITES

For an update on drugs being tested:

www.ClinicalTrials.gov
For additional information on drugs:
www.fda.gov

Other helpful Web sites include:

Centers for Disease Control	www.cdc.gov
Dr. Koop	www.drkoop.com
National Library of Medicine	www.nlm.nih.gov
Health on Net Foundation	www.hon.ch
Intelihealth	www.intelihealth.com

The following are some of the pharmaceutical Web sites that offer specific information about products mentioned in this book.

www.viagra.com
www.cialis.com
www.caverject.com
www.vivus.com
www.androgel.com
www.bayer.com

PROSTATE CANCER SURVIVOR GROUPS

Man to Man
American Cancer Society
(800) 227-2345

With over 3,400 local offices, the American Cancer Society (ACS) is committed to fighting cancer through balanced programs of research, education, patient service, advocacy, and rehabilitation.

Reading List

BOOKS ON SEXUALITY, MARRIAGE, AND COMMUNICATIONS

This is just a partial list. Other books and brochures are also available.

Gray, John. *Men Are from Mars, Women Are from Venus: A Practical Guide for Improving Communication and Getting What You Want in Your Relationship,* 1992, HarperCollins. ISBN: 006016848X.

Michael, Robert T., Edward O. Laumann, and Gina Bari Kolata. *Sex in America, A Definitive Survey.* 1995, Warner Books. ISBN: 0446671835.

Milsten, Richard, and Julian Slowinski. *The Sexual Male, Problems & Solutions.* 1999, Norton. ISBN: 0393047407.

Silbergeld, Bernie. *New Male Sexuality,* Revised Edition. 1996, Bantam Doubleday Dell. ISBN: 0553380427.

Questionnaire

Fill This Out and Take It to Your Doctor

COMPREHENSIVE QUESTIONNAIRE AND DATA FORM

This form can save you and your doctor time and help organize your visit to your doctor.

Take a few minutes to fill out this form. After completing it you will have a compilation of your personal, sexual, medical, surgical, and psychological history. You can use it to help you talk to your doctor and answer his questions, or you can simply fill it out and take it to your doctor. He or she will definitely appreciate it that you prepared this information for your visit and are ready to discuss it.

Make a copy of the completed form for your own files before taking it to your doctor. Update it often to reflect any new treatments, medications, medical conditions, insurance coverage or other changes. If the space provided is not enough, please feel free to add further information on separate pieces of paper.

DATE: _____

Part I: Personal History

Last name: _____   First name: _____ MI: _____
Date of birth: _____
Home address:
Street: _____
City:_____   State: _____ Zip: _____
Work address:
Company name:_____
Street:_____
City:_____   State: _____ Zip: _____
Home phone: (   )_____
Work phone: (   )_____
E-mail: _____

Insurance: _____
Referring doctor:_____
Occupation: _____
Years of education:_____
Other personal information:

_____

_____

Part II: Sexual History

Marital Status (circle one): Single   Married   Widowed
Divorced   Separated   Living in a relationship
Your sexual orientation (circle one):
Heterosexual   Homosexual   Bisexual
Do you have difficulty obtaining erections?   yes   no
Do you have difficulty maintaining erections until completion of
sexual activity?   yes   no

How long have you had one or both difficulties? _____

Are you satisfied with your erections?   yes   no

Has this difficulty started (circle one):   Suddenly?
Gradually?

Were there any circumstances around the onset of your erection
difficulty?   yes   no

If yes, please describe:

_____

_____

Do you wake up from sleep with erections?   yes   no

If you wake up with erections, are they rigid? yes   no

Are you able to obtain erections with:

    Foreplay: yes   no

    Masturbation: yes   no

    Sexual fantasies: yes   no

    Erotic scenes: yes   no

How would you rate your sexual desire?

strong   adequate   weak

Are you able to reach orgasm?   yes   no

Are you able to ejaculate?   yes   no

Do you have any pain with erection and/or sexual activity?

                                      yes   no

Are you satisfied with your sexual performance?   yes   no

Is your partner satisfied with your sexual performance? yes   no

Have you had any prior diagnostic evaluation of your erection
difficulty?

                                      yes   no

If yes, what was the result(s)? Please describe:

_____

_____

Have you had any prior treatment of your erection difficulty?

                                      yes   no

If yes, what was the treatment? Check all that apply and give
name of drug.

_____ Oral medication: _____

_____ Self-injection therapy: _____

_____ MUSE®

_____ Vacuum device

_____ Herbal medication: _____

_____ Hormones

_____ Penile implant

_____ Others: please describe: _____

_____

What were the result(s) of these treatments?

_____

_____

Additional comments:

_____

_____

If you are currently in a relationship with a sexual partner, how long have you been in this relationship? _____

How would you describe your relationship?

_____

_____

Do you feel sexually attracted to your partner?   yes   no

How has your sexual partner's reaction been to your erection difficulty? Please describe:

_____

_____

Does your partner have sexual difficulty?   yes   no

       If yes, please describe:

_____

_____

Part III: Medical, Surgical, Psychological Information

Height: _____   Weight: _____

Have you ever had any serious illnesses?   yes   no

Which ones?

_____

_____

Have you ever had any previous surgery?   yes   no
    List type, date:

_____

_____

Do you take medicine regularly?   yes   no
    Which ones?

_____

_____

Do you have any general allergies or allergies to medicine?
                                                         yes   no
    List and describe reaction:

_____

_____

Have you had or do you have any of the following?

    High blood pressure   yes   no
    Heart attack   yes   no
    Heart failure   yes   no
    Chest pain with rest or exercise   yes   no
    Shortness of breath   yes   no
    Ankle swelling   yes   no
    Sleeping on more than one pillow   yes   no
    Shortness of breath with rest or exercise   yes   no
    Heart murmur or mitral valve prolapse   yes   no
    Irregular heartbeat   yes   no
    Rheumatic fever   yes   no

Have you had any problems with:
    Lungs and breathing system   yes   no
    Kidneys or bladder   yes   no
    Difficulty with urination   yes   no
    Kidney failure   yes   no
    Sickle-cell disease   yes   no

Seizures	yes	no
Fainting spells or strokes	yes	no
Head, neck, or back injury	yes	no
Extreme nervousness or anxiety	yes	no
Psychiatric illness	yes	no
Diabetes	yes	no
Thyroid disease	yes	no
Hepatitis or jaundice	yes	no
Ulcers or hiatus hernia	yes	no
Glaucoma	yes	no
Hearing problems	yes	no

Please explain:

_____

_____

Have you ever had cancer?   yes   no

If yes, describe type of cancer, organ(s) involved, date of diagnosis:

_____

_____

Have you had:

Surgery for cancer	yes	no
Radiation therapy	yes	no
Chemotherapy	yes	no
Hormonal therapy	yes	no

Do you smoke?   yes   no
    How much do you smoke? _____
    How long have you smoked?_____
Do you drink alcohol?   yes   no
    How much do you drink per week?_____

Do you use marijuana, cocaine, or similar drugs?   yes   no

Part IV: ED Intensity and ED Impact Scales

ED INTENSITY SCALE

Each question has several responses. Circle the number of the response that best describes your own situations. Please be sure that you select one and only one response for each question.
Note: *The following questions should be completed only by men who have been sexually active and have attempted sexual intercourse in the past 3 months. For sexually inactive men, the questionnaire may be answered for the last period of time (3 months or longer) during which the individual was sexually active.*

1. How often were you able to get an erection during sexual activity?

Almost never or never	1
A few times (much less than half the time)	2
Sometimes (about half the time)	3
Most times (much more than half the time)	4
Almost always or always	5

2. When you had erections with sexual stimulation, how often were your erections hard enough for penetration (entering your partner)?

Almost never or never	1
A few times (much less than half the time)	2
Sometimes (about half the time)	3
Most times (much more than half the time)	4
Almost always or always	5

3. When you attempted intercourse, how often were you able to penetrate (enter) your partner?

Almost never or never	1
A few times (much less than half the time)	2
Sometimes (about half the time)	3

| Most times (much more than half the time) | 4 |
| Almost always or always | 5 |

4. During sexual intercourse, how often were you able to maintain your erection after you had penetrated (entered) your partner?

Almost never or never	1
A few times (much less than half the time)	2
Sometimes (about half the time)	3
Most times (much more than half the time)	4
Almost always or always	5

5. During sexual intercourse, how difficult was it to maintain your erection to completion of intercourse?

Extremely difficult	1
Very difficult	2
Difficult	3
Slightly difficult	4
Not difficult	5

Instructions for scoring: Add the scores for each item 1 through 5 (total possible score = 25). ED severity classification: total score 5–10 (severe ED); 11–15 (moderate ED); 16–20 (mild ED); and 21–25 (no ED or normal)

ED IMPACT (DISTRESS OR BOTHER) SCALE

If you were to spend the rest of your life with your erectile condition the way it is now, how would you feel about that?

Very dissatisfied   1
Rather dissatisfied   2
Mixed, about equally satisfied and dissatisfied   3
Rather satisfied   4
Very satisfied   5

DEPRESSION SCREENING

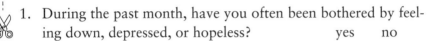

1. During the past month, have you often been bothered by feeling down, depressed, or hopeless?   yes   no

2. During the past month, have you often been bothered by little interest or pleasure in doing things?   yes   no

Part V: Physical Exam

To be filled out by your doctor, if he or she chooses:

General condition:
Weight:
Height:
HEENT:
Neck:
Chest:
Lungs:
Heart:
Abdomen:
Genitalia:
        Penis:
        Scrotum:
        Testicles:

Digital rectal exam:
Perineal exam:
Neurological exam:
Extremities:
Musculoskeletal:
Skin:
Other:

Part VI: Lab Tests (Optional)

Testosterone (date: /   /   ):
Fasting blood sugar (date: /   /   ):
Cholesterol (date: /   /   ):
Other lab tests (date: /   /   ):

Part VII: Additional Tests (Optional)

Penile Doppler ultrasound (date: /   /   ):
RigiScan (date: /   /   ):
Other tests (date: /   /   ):

Index